Care Trajectory Management

Care Trajectory Management

Foundations in the Organising Work of Nurses

DAVINA ALLEN, RN, BA (HONS), PHD

Professor of Healthcare Work and Organisation
School of Healthcare Sciences
Cardiff University
Cardiff, United Kingdom

ELSEVIER

ISBN: 978-0-443-10753-5

Content Strategist: Andrae Akeh
Content Project Manager: Tapajyoti Chaudhuri
Cover Design: Amy L. Buxton
Marketing Manager: Deborah J. Watkins

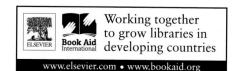

Working together to grow libraries in developing countries

www.elsevier.com • www.bookaid.org

Printed in India
Last digit is the print number: 9 8 7 6 5 4 3 2 1

CONTENTS

BBC	British Broadcasting Corporation
BG	Blood glucose
BP	Blood pressure
COPD	Chronic obstructive pulmonary disease
CT scan	Computed tomography scan
CTM	Care trajectory management
CVA	Cerebral vascular accident
DNAR	Do not attempt resuscitation
GTN	Glyceryl trinitrate
IM	Intramuscular
IV	Intravenous
IVI	Intravenous infusion
MDT	Multidisciplinary team
MSU	Midstream specimen of urine
NHS	National Health Service
NMC	Nursing & Midwifery Council
OT	Occupational therapist
PE	Pulmonary embolism
RCN	Royal College of Nursing
TMT	Translational Mobilisation Theory
TTH	Tablets to take home
UK	United Kingdom
UKCC	United Kingdom Central Council for Nursing, Midwifery and Health Visiting
US	United States
VQ scan	Ventilation (V) and quantity (Q) of perfusion scan
WHO	World Health Organization

Davina Allen is a sociologist and nurse academic. She is Professor of Healthcare work and organisation at Cardiff University, Wales, and Professor II at Norwegian University of Science and Technology, Gjøvik, Norway. She has been researching nursing and the caring division of labour, healthcare delivery and organisation, and service improvement technologies for over 30 years. Her work includes foundational ethnographic studies of healthcare organisation, a long-standing programme of research on the work of nurses and large-scale applied interdisciplinary research projects on the development and evaluation of improvement interventions.

ACKNOWLEDGEMENTS

This book is derived from empirical research on the organisational elements of the nursing role, discussed in my book *The Invisible Work of Nurses: Hospitals, Organisation and Healthcare* of 2015. In the intervening period, the ideas outlined in the original study have been advanced through work with Carl May, with whom I developed Translational Mobilisation Theory; conversations with Heather Strange, Alison Evans and nurses from Cardiff and Vale University Health Board, which helped to keep my thinking grounded in practice; and collaboration with Aud Uhlen Obstfelder, Anne Marie Rafferty and Mary Ellen Purkis to specify strategies for integrating preparation for care trajectory management into nurse education.

Aud Uhlen Obstfelder and Alison Evans, generously provided feedback on drafts of the text. In the conclusion of The Invisible Work of Nurses, I highlighted the changes to education, policy and practice required for the organisational aspects of nursing work to be formally recognised. While these changes are substantial, my hope is that this text will be an important resource in progressing this agenda. Extracts from the original study are reproduced here for illustrative purposes by permission of Taylor & Francis Group.

Davina Allen

Cardiff, UK

December 2023

My discovery, as a patient first on a medical service and later in surgery, is that the institution is held together, glued together, enabled to function as an organism, by the nurses and by nobody else.

Thomas (1983)

The decision was made—we had to establish a cohort unit. Well, when you put these ideas down on paper and have it all figured out, it seems to work fine. But the moment they [the board] said 'Go for it!', well, I can still see the look in the eyes of the physician who thought, 'Okay then…' [clueless]. But also, the look in the eyes of the chief nurse, like 'Okay!' [decisive]. The chief nurse just took care of it, and in a blink of an eye, it was all set: the COVID unit was set up, everyone knew what to do, and the materials had been delivered. And the appreciation of the physician, who hadn't known what to do….To me, that moment revealed a huge difference in expertise. The physician might know everything about the disease, about the treatment, and what is known at that time. But organising care for a patient is a different profession, a different and true craft I'd say.

Nurse and secretary of the Board of Directors,
February 2021; Kuijper et al. (2022, p. 1306)

What Is Care Trajectory Management and Why Does It Matter?

This book is written for nurses wishing to deepen their understanding, knowledge and skills in care trajectory management. Care trajectory management is a relatively new concept, which refers to the well-established, but largely invisible, organising nursing practices that hold together patient care (Allen, 2018a).

Healthcare is complex. It is a work of many hands (Aveling et al., 2016), which involves numerous professions, technicians and support workers, who have distinctive skills, knowledge and expertise. It spans different departments and organisations, each with their singular operating models, governance processes and funding mechanisms. It includes a wide range of technologies extending from everyday applications, devices and medicines, through to sophisticated innovations in telemedicine, artificial intelligence and robotics. It is also intrinsically unpredictable work. Troubled bodies and unsettled minds can be challenging to understand, and they may act in unexpected ways, particularly if the person has more than one condition. Interventions to address a problem in one part of the body can create difficulties elsewhere, the management of which may in turn bring its own complications. The contexts of care are also inherently turbulent. Whether in the home or the hospital, the care of individuals must be balanced with the care of others, and because healthcare systems have little control over demand, case mix is subject to churn (Duffield et al., 2007; Melia, 1979). Arrangements for homecare and community support must be acceptable to the patient and their family, and sufficiently flexible to accommodate shifting needs.

Complex systems of work, like healthcare, have centrifugal tendencies; they pull apart, and the elements that make up an individual's care do not hold together on their own. Action is necessary to ensure that patients receive the right care, in the right place, at the right time, by the right person, with the right outcome. This is no mean feat, and it is nurses who fulfil this function. Nurses make it their business to know everything that is going on. They monitor and make sense of patients' ongoing care, they respond to contingencies and anticipate needs, they facilitate communication within the healthcare team, they take responsibility for ensuring that materials and technologies are available to support clinical procedures, and they mobilise and coordinate action. It is these organising practices that are conceptualised here as care trajectory management. Care trajectory management is important work; it enables healthcare organisations to function despite the unpredictable qualities of the system and makes an essential contribution to the quality and safety of patient care.

Important work though it may be, care trajectory management is not a formally recognised component of the nursing role. At one level, this reflects nursing's strategy for improving its status and bargaining power in society, in which the profession's claim to expertise has been expressed almost exclusively in terms of its care-giving function (Allen, 2001; Armstrong, 1983). At another level, it reflects the progressive influence of general management approaches to the challenges of organisation in healthcare systems (Strong and Robinson, 1990; Traynor, 1999). Thus, while often referred to colloquially as the 'glue' within healthcare systems, for the last 50 years or so, the nursing contribution to the organisation of patient care has been largely taken for granted. In the past, student nurses received limited explicit preparation for this aspect of their work, with expertise in care trajectory management typically built up after graduation. And despite its ubiquity, nursing has not had a vocabulary with which to explain, describe or study this aspect of professional practice. Not only does this impact on the visibility of the nursing contribution to healthcare in policy circles and public perception, but it also makes it difficult for experienced nurses to share their knowledge to facilitate the learning of others or use their expertise to advance practice, either through research or quality improvement initiatives.

Ensuring the quality and safety of healthcare is a global priority. In this context, there is a growing realisation of the need to formally acknowledge the organisational components of the nursing role (Butler et al., 2006; Hope, 2004; Noordegraaf, 2015; Nursing and Midwifery Council, 2018; Smith et al., 2021). This is essential to guide recruitment and selection (Noordegraaf, 2015), to integrate care trajectory management into nurse education (Allen et al., 2019), to safeguard nurses' well-being (Smith et al., 2021) and to ensure that the profession can realise its leadership potential in healthcare systems (DiMattio, 2015). This textbook is designed to facilitate these aims by providing theoretical and conceptual resources to enable nurses to describe, explain and study this safety critical component of their work.

What Is the Research Evidence That Informs the Theories and Concepts of Care Trajectory Management?

This book is research led and evidence based. It is underpinned by theories, concepts and concrete resources derived from in-depth qualitative research which for the first time examined the real-world practices involved in care trajectory management. *The Invisible Work of Nurses* (Allen, 2015) study was carried out in a large tertiary hospital in the United Kingdom (UK) and was designed to shine a light on the organisational dimensions of nursing work. I shadowed 40 nurses in the adult care context and observed their work and discussed their practice. The nurses who participated in the research all had frontline clinical responsibilities; they were not nurse managers. Essential as this work is, I was interested in the patient-facing aspects of nurses' organising work, rather than formal management roles. It is the knowledge and skills nurses develop in managing patient trajectories of care which provide the foundations for the nursing contribution to the organisation of services at other levels within the healthcare system. The nurses included in the study were drawn from a wide range of roles to capture the full spectrum of their organising work. The selection of participants was informed by an expert reference group of nurses from education, research, service and policy. Each nurse was shadowed for approximately 8 hours, over several occasions.

The research was informed by several sociological theories: practice theory (Nicolini, 2012), actor network theory (Latour, 2005) and the negotiated order perspective (Strauss et al., 1963). You will learn more about these later in this text. For the purposes of the original study, they informed my approach to data generation, directing attention to what nurses did in organising patient care and the tools they used for this purpose, the knowledge and skills that underpinned nurses' organising practices and the circumstances that made their organising work necessary. I recorded my observations as handwritten fieldnotes in a notebook, documenting as precisely as possible activities and dialogue as these happened. After each period of observation, I word-processed the fieldnotes, fleshing out any missing details from memory. The word-processed files were then uploaded into qualitative data analysis software, which was used to apply electronic codes to sections of the data to enable retrieval of areas of interest for the purposes of analysis. I analysed my data as I went along and shared my ideas with research participants to assess whether my interpretations made sense from their perspective. Thus, while informed by sociological theory, the final analysis was also embedded in the perspectives of nurses.

The research revealed that the need for care trajectory management arises because of the complexity and unpredictability of healthcare work, in which the organisation of care is often emergent and responsive rather than linear and planned. While a multiplicity of formal structures and procedures exist for the purposes of organising activity—care pathways, checklists, referral processes, guidelines, risk assessments and standards—on their own these are insufficient to ensure patient care is coordinated. Far from following a managed pathway through the service, for much of the time the diverse elements of an individual's care are loosely coupled and understanding of the patient is fragmented across the healthcare team. The research highlighted the central role of nurses in generating order from this complexity to hold together patient care. Drawing on actor network theory, I argued that nurses are the 'obligatory passage points' in healthcare systems. An obligatory passage point is an essential element in a network of action through which all activity must pass, rather like the narrow end of a funnel. And while nurses are not typically identified in formal policies as the primary actors in healthcare systems, in the real world barely anything happens in healthcare that does not pass through the hands (or brain) of a nurse.

> [N]urses are the means for bringing together and keeping apart the various heterogenous entities to accomplish everyday service delivery. They make the connections across occupational, departmental, and organisational boundaries and mediate the 'needs' of individuals with the 'needs' of populations. Not only is this work an essential driver of action, it operates as a powerful countervailing force to the centrifugal tendencies inherent in healthcare organisations which, for all their gloss of order and rationality are in reality very loose arrangements.
>
> (With permission from Taylor & Francis Group. Allen, D., 2015. The Invisible Work of Nurses: Hospitals, Organisation and Healthcare. Routledge, London and New York, p. 136.)

Since completion of the empirical study, further work has been undertaken to specify the competencies that underpin care trajectory management (Allen et al., 2019) and generate the theories and concepts you will learn about in this text (Allen, 2018a, 2018b; Allen and May, 2017). If you would like to know more about the original research, please go to the website https://theinvisible-workofnurses.co.uk; more detailed accounts are available in the suggestions for further reading listed at the end of this section.

About This Book

This is the first ever textbook about care trajectory management. It is both a theoretical and a practical resource. While the concepts and theories of care trajectory management are new in nursing, they build on a substantial body of sociological theory and research extending over many years. Key ideas that inform this text are represented in summative frameworks to facilitate their application to nursing practice, but I have made a deliberate decision to share and explain the intellectual origins of these new ways of thinking to facilitate deep understanding. While this book cannot teach you how to *do* care trajectory management, it is intended to inform practice.

Throughout the text, theories and concepts are illustrated with concrete examples. Some of these have been developed for learning purposes, but many are derived from observational studies of everyday healthcare work. Key learning points are reinforced through practical exercises, designed to be undertaken for the purposes of private study, but which can be easily adapted for joint learning. An online downloadable Care Trajectory Management Workbook is available to help you organise and record your learning (see Evolve website).

While the theory and practice of care trajectory management form the core of the book, in contextualising these ideas, the text ranges far and wide. Care trajectory management is examined in the context of the history of nursing's professional development, and the critical debates that have shaped, and continue to shape, societal understanding of nursing work and nurses' professional identity. The text also explores the relationship of care trajectory management with emerging approaches to healthcare quality and safety and organising in conditions of complexity. By reflecting on where nursing has come from, and scanning future horizons, a clearer sense of professional direction can be advanced.

This is an unusual text in that it is aimed at experienced and newly qualified nurses and students. If you are an experienced nurse who has not received formal preparation for the care trajectory management role, it is intended to better equip you to explain, describe and apply your expertise, as clinician, mentor, educator, manager and professional leader. If you are a newly qualified nurse, it is designed to help you adapt to the demands of the registrant role and plan your professional development. If you are a student nurse, it is designed to foster an understanding of care trajectory management and its contribution to patient care to maximise learning from practice placements, increase competencies at the point of qualification and accelerate your professional development thereafter. Through these dual mechanisms, the ambition is to better prepare future generations of nurses for care trajectory management and provide a language to articulate this component of practice, to optimise the profession's global contribution to the quality and safety of patient care, increase the visibility of this work in healthcare systems and inform public understanding of the nursing role.

The text is organised into two sections. Section I describes and explains the professional, practice and policy context for care trajectory management. Chapter 1 traces the history of organising work in nursing and examines the changes in contemporary healthcare systems that have led to an increase in the work involved in the organisation and coordination of patient care. It also considers the contribution of concepts and theories for making organising work visible and enabling nursing knowledge to be shared. Chapter 2 introduces the two core concepts that form the backbone for this text: care trajectory and care trajectory management. It explores the implications of viewing patient care processes as trajectories rather than pathways and considers the relationship of care trajectory management to the wider aspects of the nursing role. Chapter 3 analyses the conditions that make care trajectory management necessary and the features of healthcare work that give rise to this complexity. Chapter 4 focuses on different approaches to organising healthcare. It explores the differences between rational–linear and emergent organisation, the interrelationship between these approaches in everyday practice and their implications for care trajectory management. Chapters 5 and 6 consider the importance of care trajectory management for healthcare systems. Chapter 5 examines why care trajectory management matters to patients through an in-depth exploration of the international research evidence on the relationship between care coordination and the quality and safety of patient care. Chapter 6 considers why care trajectory management matters for nursing. It critically examines the reasons for the invisibility of the organisational elements of nursing work and explains, through empirical examples, why formal recognition of care trajectory management is important for the everyday work of individual nurses and the ability of the wider profession to realise its contribution to healthcare systems.

Section II is concerned with the theories and concepts that underpin care trajectory management and their application to nursing practice. Chapter 7 introduces the Translational Mobilisation Theory (TMT) and explores how its domain assumptions offer new ways of seeing healthcare for the purposes of care trajectory management. Chapter 8 builds on Chapter 7 to focus on the core components of TMT. Together, these chapters provide conceptual resources which describe and explain how activities are organised in complex systems of work. Having established these theoretical foundations, Chapter 9 introduces the Care Trajectory Management Framework, which offers a structure with which to describe and explain care trajectory management practices. Chapter 10, the final chapter of the text, brings these insights together. It summarises the skills and competencies that underpin care trajectory management and applies these to practice through a series of exercises based on real-world scenarios.

The book is designed to be read sequentially, at least initially. Each chapter builds foundations for subsequent chapters and includes a summative exercise to enable you to assess your learning, before progressing further. Once you are familiar with the main tenets of care trajectory management, it is possible to dip in and out of the materials for reference purposes or to consolidate your learning. Throughout the book, there are case studies and exercises which presuppose some practice experience. This is important to bear in mind when planning programmes of study. Beyond the main body of the text, each chapter includes the following features:

- Chapter outline
- Learning outcomes
- Definitions
- Interesting facts
- Case studies
- Reflections on practice
- Exercises
- Summary of key learning
- References
- Quick quiz
- Annotated suggested reading
- Indicative answers for key exercises

These features are designed to support independent study and enable you to navigate the sections relevant to your needs. Experienced nurses, for example, may wish to skip some of the practice exercises, but undertake suggested further reading designed to encourage critical reflection and develop in-depth understanding. Nurse lecturers may wish to supplement the materials in this text with additional practice scenarios to support student learning. Learning is a lifelong process in which much of the action takes place at the boundary between formal study and workplace experience. The aim of this text is to sharpen the senses in relation to the care trajectory management function and provide practical and cognitive resources to support continual professional development along the pathway to expert practice.

References

Allen, D., 2001. The Changing Shape of Nursing Practice: The Role of Nurses in the Hospital Division of Labour. Routledge, London and New York.

Allen, D., 2015. The Invisible Work of Nurses: Hospitals, Organisation and Healthcare. Routledge, London and New York.

Allen, D., 2018a. Care trajectory management: a conceptual framework for formalising emergent organisation in nursing practice. J. Nurs. Manag. 27 (1), 4–9.

Allen, D., 2018b. Translational Mobilisation Theory: a new paradigm for understanding the organisational components of nursing work. Int. J. Nurs. Stud. 79 (March 2018), 36–42.

Allen, D. and May, C., 2017. Organizing practice and practicing organization: towards an outline of translational mobilization theory. Sage Open. 7 (2). doi: 10.1177/2158244017707993.

Allen, D., Purkis, M.E., Rafferty, A.M., Obstfelder, A., 2019. Integrating preparation for care trajectory management into nurse education: competencies and pedagogical strategies. Nurs. Inq 26 (3), e12289. doi: 10.1111/nin.12289.

Armstrong, D., 1983. The fabrication of nurse-patient relationships. Soc. Sci. Med. 17 (8), 457–460.

Aveling, E., Parker, M., Dixon-Woods, M., 2016. What is the role of individual accountability in patient safety? A multi-site ethnographic study. Sociol. Health Illn. 38 (2), 216–232.

Butler, M., Scott, P.A., Hyde, A., Treacy, P.M., 2006. Towards a nursing minimum data set for Ireland: making Irish nursing visible. J. Adv. Nurs. 55 (3), 364–375.

DiMattio, M.J.K., 2015. A view from the board room. Nurs. Outlook. 63 (5), 533–536.

Duffield, C.M. & University of Technology, Sydney, Centre for Health Services Management & NSW Health, 2007. Glueing It Together: Nurses, Their Work Environment and Patient Safety, Final Report. Centre for Health Services Management, Sydney, Australia.

Hope, H.A., 2004. Working conditions of the nursing workforce: excerpts from a policy roundtable at Academy Health's 2003 Annual Research Meeting. Health Serv. Res. 39 (3), 445–461.

Kuijper, S., Felder, M., Bal, R., Wallenburg, I., 2022. Assembling care: how nurses organise care in uncharted territory and in times of pandemic. Sociol. Health Illn. 44 (8), 1305–1323.

Latour, B., 2005. Reassembling the Social: An Introduction to Actor-Network-Theory. Oxford University Press, Oxford.

Melia, K.M., 1979. A sociological approach to the analysis of nursing work. J. Adv. Nurs. 4, 57–67.

Nicolini, D., 2012. Practice Theory, Work and Organization: An Introduction. Oxford University Press, Oxford.

Noordegraaf, M., 2015. Hybrid professionalism and beyond: (new) forms of public professionalism in changing organizational and societal contexts. J. Prof. Organ. 2 (2), 187–206.

Nursing and Midwifery Council, 2018. Future Nurse: Standards of Proficiency for Registered Nurses. London. Nursing and Midwifery Council. https://www.nmc.org.uk/standards/standards-for-nurses/standards-of-proficiency-for-registered-nurses/ (Accessed 8 December 2022).

Smith, P., Brennan, G.K., Mansilla Castillo, D., Adhikari, R., 2021. Perspectives: this house believes that a natural facet of nursing work is that it depletes nurses' wellbeing. J. Res. Nurs. 26 (3), 264–271. doi:10.1177/17449871211014021.

Strauss, A., Schatzman, L., Bucher, R., Ehrlich, D., Sabshin, M., 1963. The hospital and its negotiated order. In: Freidson, E. (Ed.), The Hospital in Modern Society. Free Press of Glencoe, New York, pp. 147–169.

Strong, P., Robinson, J., 1990. The NHS Under New Management. Open University Press, Buckingham.

Thomas, L., 1983. The Youngest Science: Notes of a Medicine Watcher. Viking Press, New York.

Traynor, M., 1999. Managerialism and Nursing: Beyond Oppression and Profession. Routledge, London.

Suggested Reading

Allen, D., 2015. The Invisible Work of Nurses: Hospitals, Organisation and Healthcare. Routledge, London.
This text reports on the full study and includes detailed information on the research methods, theoretical framework, rich ethnographic descriptions of nursing work and consideration of the implications of the research for nursing and healthcare policy and practice.

Allen, D., 2014. Reconceptualising holism within the contemporary nursing mandate: from individual to organisational relationships. Soc. Sci. Med. 119, 131–138.
This paper draws on the findings from *The Invisible Work of Nurses* to argue for an extension of the concept of holism to include organisational as well as nurse–patient relationships as the basis for the nursing's scope of professional practice.

What Is Care Trajectory Management and Why Does It Matter?

Section I introduces care trajectory management and considers its importance for policy and practice. It traces the evolution of organising work in the nursing role, the features of modern healthcare systems which have given rise to the requirement for care trajectory management and the reasons for its invisibility. It describes the concepts of care trajectory and care trajectory management and explains how together these facilitate understanding of the complex nursing practices involved in coordinating and organising patient care. The contribution of care trajectory management to healthcare quality and safety and the policy and practical implications of its continued invisibility are reviewed to develop the case for formal recognition of care trajectory management in the contemporary nursing role.

Concepts and Making the Invisible, Visible

LEARNING OUTCOMES

At the end of this chapter, you will be able to:
- Describe the historical changes to the organisational component of nursing work
- Explain the importance of concepts and theories for professional practice

Introduction

Care trajectory management is a new concept, which has been coined to refer to the work that nurses do in organising patient care processes. This work makes a central contribution to healthcare quality and safety and the resilience of organisations, but for too long, it has been a taken for granted rather than formally sanctioned as an element of the nursing role. One important aim of this book is to deepen the understanding of care trajectory management and provide concepts and theories with which to describe and explain this component of nursing practice in order that the profession can realise fully its potential. In the first step of this process, this chapter traces the history and evolution of the organisational component of nursing work and explores its contribution to contemporary healthcare systems. It describes the factors that have increased the volume and complexity of organising work in nursing practice and considers how theories and concepts have value in making visible this invisible component of the nursing role.

A Short History of the Organisational Component of Nursing Work

Since the emergence of nursing as a formally recognised occupation in the mid-19th century, nursing work has always included an organisational component. Despite the dominant image in popular culture of Florence Nightingale as a bedside nurse (Fig. 1.1), her contribution to

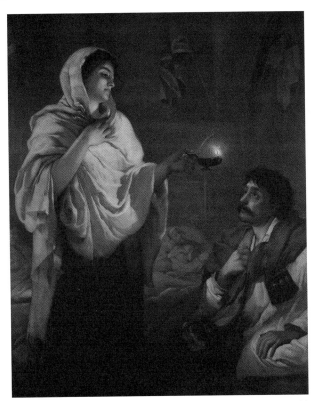

Fig. 1.1 Crimean War: Florence Nightingale with her lamp at a patient's bedside. (From Henrietta Rae, 1891; Wellcome Collection Creative Commons Licence CC-BY.)

healthcare had as much to do with improving the organisation of services and enhancing sanitary conditions as with directly attending to the comfort of patients (Dingwall et al., 1988).

> *Bad sanitary, bad architectural, and bad administrative arrangements often make it impossible to nurse. But the art of nursing ought to include such arrangements as alone make what I understand by nursing possible.*
>
> Nightingale (1860/1969, p. 8)

Nineteenth century nursing was primarily concerned with creating the environments to foster health and healing. This entailed managing the physical setting for reasons related to treatment, care and hygiene, but also to make the care of many patients possible within the context of related administrative structures (Allen et al., 2019). The organisational component of nursing work at this time included traditional household activities, moving heavy equipment, walking endless corridors, as well as making the arrangements for putting into use new technologies for diagnosis and treatment (Sandelowski, 2000).

In the intervening period, healthcare work has been transformed by advances in science and technology, changes to the structure and organisation of services and the impact of demographic trends and shifting disease patterns on patient populations. At the beginning of the 19th century, the primary cause of mortality was infectious diseases, and medical practice was focused on symptom management. Paid healthcare work was undertaken primarily by doctors and nurses, and a typical hospital would have looked more like a convalescent ward (Dingwall and Allen, 2001).

Today, hospital populations are characterised by high levels of acuity, complexity and rapid throughput. There has been a growth in the prevalence of long-term conditions, with many people living with comorbidities. Specialist healthcare services and professions have proliferated, increasing the difficulty of care coordination. Owing to new medical technologies, changes in family structures and redistributions of healthcare work, many people are now cared for in the community and depend on complex and finely balanced arrangements for condition management and ongoing support (Bjornsdottir, 2018; Exley and Allen, 2007; Hannigan and Allen, 2013; Melby et al., 2018).

Changes in the content and organisation of healthcare have transformed the work of nurses. Many fundamental aspects of patient care now are performed by support staff under the supervision of registrants, while the complexity of the clinical components of nursing work has increased. Nurses now carry out a range of specialist interventions, such as renal dialysis, chemotherapy, cognitive behavioural therapy and assertive outreach (Stephenson, 2018), and work in a variety of advanced practitioner and specialist roles.

Alongside these changes in clinical nursing care, there has also been an increase in the volume and complexity of the organisational component of nursing work (Furaker, 2009; Michel et al., 2017). While the profession has divested itself of the housekeeping tasks associated with the 19th century nursing role, contemporary nurses remain responsible for healthcare environments, through standard setting, audit, quality improvement and workforce management, activities typically led by nurse managers. One of the most significant changes in the work of nurses over the last century, however, has been the progressive expansion of activities related to the organisation and coordination of patient care and treatment.

In 2004 I carried out a review of observational studies of nursing work published in the English language between 1993 and 2003 (Allen, 2004). The paper was an invited contribution to a special edition of *Nursing Inquiry*, marking the 10th anniversary of the journal. The question driving the review was: What do nurses do when they go to work? Observational studies are well suited to answering this question as they offer a window on to real-world practices, revealing what nurses do, rather than what they say they do. The review included 54 publications: 8 books, 10 book chapters and 36 journal articles. The studies were carried out in hospital, community and nursing home settings in the UK (35), United States (7), Canada (5), Australia (4), Sweden (2) and Belgium (1). My purpose was not to report on all aspects of the included studies, but to draw out and analyse the insights offered by this body of work on the shape and content of nursing practice. Inspired by the ideas of the sociologist E.C. Hughes (1984), who conceptualised occupational roles as bundles of tasks, I identified eight bundles of activity comprising nursing work (Box 1.1). Together these highlighted the centrality of organising work in the contemporary nursing role.

Healthcare is a collective activity, but whether it is in the hospital, care home or community, it is nurses that have most continuing contact with patients and families. It is because of this singular occupational niche that nurses fulfil an important role in coordinating activity.

Field studies indicate that in modern healthcare systems the core nursing function is to mediate different agenda, articulate the work of different care providers around individual patients, and fabricate patient identities from diverse information sources. It is nurses who reconcile the requirements of healthcare organisations with those of patients and constitute and prioritise needs in response to available resources. It is nurses who broker, interpret, translate, and communicate clinical, social, and organisational information in ways that are consequential for patient diagnoses and outcomes. It is nurses who work flexibly to blur their jurisdictional boundaries with those of others […] to ensure continuity of care. In fulfilling these roles, it is nurses who weave together the many facets of the service and create order in a fast flowing and turbulent work environment.

Allen (2004, pp. 278–279)

> **BOX 1.1** ■ **Eight Bundles of Nursing Activity Identified in a Review of Observational Studies of Nursing Work**
>
> **Managing Multiple Agenda**
> The work of nurses in mediating the different agenda that shape healthcare systems.
>
> **Circulating Patients**
> The work of nurses in managing patient throughput.
>
> **Bringing the Individual Into the Organisation**
> The work of nurses in individualising care in the application of standards and routines.
>
> **Managing the Work of Others**
> The work of nurses in organising the activities of other members of the healthcare team, in particular junior doctors.
>
> **Mediating Occupational Boundaries**
> The work that nurses do in working flexibly to ensure that care does not fall through the gaps in formal role descriptions.
>
> **Obtaining, Fabricating, Interpreting and Communicating Information**
> The work of nurses in making sense of patient care and managing information flows between the healthcare team.
>
> **Maintaining a Record**
> The work of nurses in creating and maintaining clinical documentation.
>
> **Prioritising Care and Rationing Resources**
> The work of nurses in balancing the needs of individuals with the needs of whole patient populations within available capacity.
>
> ---
>
> With permission from Allen, D., 2004. Re-reading nursing and re-writing practice: towards an empirically based reformulation of the nursing mandate. Nurs. Inquiry. 11(4), 271–283.

Despite its ubiquity across a variety of international care environments, organising work is not formally recognised as a core element of the nursing role (Allen, 2004, 2015). On the contrary, it is regularly implicated in professional and policy debates about increased bureaucracy in healthcare systems, where it is framed as illegitimate work which takes nurses away from their rightful work with patients. For example, in 2013, the BBC reported on the findings of a survey undertaken by the UK Royal College of Nursing (RCN) which claimed that nurses are 'drowning in a sea of paperwork' (BBC, 2013). The poll of 6000 nurses claimed that 17.3% of their hours was spent on paperwork, with most reporting that it was stopping them providing direct patient care. Commenting on the survey findings, the then RCN general secretary Peter Carter said, 'These figures prove what a shocking amount of a nurse's time is being wasted on unnecessary paperwork and bureaucracy […] patients want their nurses by the bedside, not ticking boxes'. Andrew Gwynne, shadow health minister concurred, arguing, 'Now form-filling is taking nurses away from their patients for longer and longer'.

These arguments are not without foundation. It is obvious that with a finite workforce, nurses must make judgements about how to use their time and energy. This is a zero-sum game which will involve difficult trade-offs, many of which present professional dilemmas, particularly in the context of persistent nursing workforce shortages. It is also the case that in recent years, there has been a monumental increase in the administrative burdens of contemporary healthcare systems, and as you will have probably experienced, not all of this 'polyformacy' (Allen, 2017) adds value (Box 1.2). But to focus on the difficulties of prioritising nursing activities and excessive bureaucracy is to focus on the symptoms, rather than the underlying issue, which is the growing

---

BOX 1.2 ■ Use of Standard Risk Screening and Assessment Forms to Prevent Harm to Older People in Australian Hospitals: A Mixed-Methods Study

Standard risk screening and assessment forms are frequently used in strategies to prevent harm to older people in hospitals. But little is known about good practice for their use. Redley and Raggatt (2017) carried out a mixed-methods study on risk assessment tools in the care of older people in Victoria Australia. The methods included:

1. a cross-sectional audit of the standard risk screening and assessment forms used to assess older people at 11 health services in 2015; and
2. nine focus groups with a purposively selected sample of 69 participants at nine health services.

Paper or electronic versions of all the standard risk assessment forms used in the care of older people were collected from the key site contact. The number of items on forms, preventable harms assessed and sources of duplication were analysed and described. Analysis of focus group data identified themes explaining issues commonly affecting how health services used the forms.

A key finding from the study was the sheer volume of risk assessment tools that were identified in the 11 health services—52 in total—and the concomitant burdens these generated for staff. At one level, there was a *workload burden* associated with the volume of forms staff had to complete. The workload was most pronounced during the admission process, with assessments taking between 40 minutes and 2 hours. Many of the tools in use overlapped and there was considerable duplication of effort. At another level, there were *cognitive burdens* associated with the challenges of locating and interpreting information collected across multiple forms, which were often completed in professional silos. Participants noted that busy and/or inexperienced staff were primarily concerned with completing the forms within the prescribed timeframe, rather than using the information to inform clinical judgments about the patient's care requirements. They also reported that risks highlighted by the assessments were not recognised. Reviewing the tools in use, the authors also identified gaps in assessment of several preventable harms: unresolved pain, incontinences and cognitive impairments.

The authors identified that an important driver for the selection and use of risk assessment tools in the 11 health services in the study was the requirement for accreditation with Australia's National Safety Quality Health Service Standards. It has become increasingly common for external agencies to impose such requirements on organisations. Redley and Raggatt report that while quality assurance processes incentivised compliance with the risk assessment *documentation*, completion of the risk assessment did not necessarily lead to *action* to mitigate any of the risks that had been identified.

The authors conclude that frontline staff require support to make complex decisions about interventions to reduce harm in older people, but that this is not facilitated by standardised risk assessment forms. Existing forms need to be streamlined to enable comprehensive interdisciplinary assessments, and quality assurance monitoring needs to shift from a focus on compliance with risk assessments to evaluating interventions that are effective in mitigating risk.

Redley, B., Raggatt, M., 2017. Use of standard risk screening and assessment forms to prevent harm to older people in Australian hospitals: a mixed methods study. BMJ Qual. Saf. 26, 704–713.

---

requirement for coordination work in contemporary healthcare systems, failures of which have catastrophic impacts on the quality and safety of patient care.

> *Western health care practices are currently far from effective, efficient, patient-centred, safe, timely, and equitable – however exactly defined – not so much because of the failings of individual health care workers, but because of a lack of coordination of their individual activities. Work around individual patient trajectories is fragmented because of intra- and interorganizational borders that have much relation with the organizations' and professions' histories, but little with the needs of patients. Tasks are not aligned; organizational routines do not articulate with each other; information is not shared.*

Timmermans and Berg (2003, p. 202)

It is this challenge that makes the organisational component of nursing practice necessary, and which underlines the importance of developing the conceptual resources to make visible this safety critical function.

Making the Invisible, Visible: Why Concepts Matter for Nursing Practice

Theory gets a lot of flak in nursing. It is often depicted as an esoteric matter unconnected to the material concerns of clinical practice. Academic nurses, in turn, are portrayed as living in ivory towers, far removed from the realities of nursing work (Webb, 2002). This ethos of anti-intellectualism has a lengthy history in the profession. Nursing has long been understood as character-based moral work (Gordon and Nelson, 2006) and an extension of an individual's natural caring qualities rather than a highly skilled practice requiring the acquisition of specialist knowledge, critical thinking and analytic skills. Despite the profound changes in the complexity of nursing practice previously described, this archetype endures: nursing is regularly portrayed as an exclusively practical occupation, in which doing is privileged over thinking, and care is privileged over science (Garcia and Qureshi, 2022). In the 1990s, the Project 2000 reform of nurse education in the UK, which was designed to strengthen preregistration preparation for practice, was met with derision by some prominent commentators (Box 1.3). Similarly, it was the academic foundations of nursing work that were targeted in the questions that were raised in the context of the UK Mid-Staffordshire care scandal, in which graduate nurses were accused of being 'too posh to wash' (Hayter, 2013) and which, at the time of writing, have resurfaced in discussions about the nursing workforce shortage in the UK.

Ambivalence about theory can also be found *within* the profession and is reflected in debates about the challenges practitioners experience in integrating knowledge learnt in an academic

---

BOX 1.3 ■ Anti-intellectualism in Public Perceptions of Nursing Work

Project 2000 (UKCC, 1987) was designed to strengthen the preregistration preparation of nurses in the UK in the 1990s. Before this time, nurse education was tied to hospital-based schools of nursing, student nurses were employed by the local health authority, and the nursing qualification was not a recognised academic standard.

The Project 2000 reforms relocated nurse education to higher education institutes, and academic skills were to be valued and rewarded by a Diploma, a formally accredited educational standard. Learners were accorded supernumerary status in practice, rather than being included as part of the workforce. The aim of the Project 2000 reforms was to produce 'knowledgeable doers' who could practice in a range of settings.

Project 2000 was rolled out across the UK throughout the 1990s, but by the end of the decade, there was mounting public and professional concern about the new model of nurse education. What is of interest for current purposes is not the success or otherwise of Project 2000, but the gendered and anti-intellectualist terms through which criticism of the reforms was articulated.

Nigella Lawson, writing in *The Times*, a leading national newspaper, argued that the reforms were misguided because they prevented 'natural [but not academic] nurses from pursuing a nursing career' and that the Project 2000 curriculum was an inadequate preparation for the practical demands of the job. She concludes that nursing 'is an honourable, worthy job; pretending it needs academic status to give it respectability is blundering offensive and silly'. Similar tropes are rehearsed by Richard Horton, then editor of the leading medical journal *The Lancet*, who argued that 'by turning their work into a science akin to medicine [nurses] risk displacing plain and simple (and decidedly non-scientific) caring'.

With permission from Taylor & Francis Group. Allen, D., Lyne, P., 2006. How did we get there? In: Allen, D., Lyne, P. (Eds.), The Reality of Nursing Research: Politics, Practices and Processes. Routledge, London and New York, pp. 12–24.
UKCC, 1987. Project 2000: The Final Proposals. UKCC, London.

environment with real-world nursing. Many early models of nursing were driven by the desire of nurse academics to develop a distinctive knowledge base which differentiated nursing from medicine (Allen, 2001; Dingwall, 1974). These were typically the product of desk-based theorising rather than empirical research, and often a poor fit with everyday nursing practice (Nelson and Gordon, 2006; Rolfe, 1993; Thorn, 2022). Despite the subsequent advances in nursing research, the so-called theory–practice gap has remained a live issue for over 40 years. But theory is only one of the many factors that contribute to this complex educational problem, which also include the structure and organisation of nurse education (Landers, 2008), workplace cultures (Sharif and Masoumi, 2005), practice constraints (Maben et al., 2006; Ousey and Gallagher, 2007), systems of mentorship (Myall et al., 2008) and the relationship between nursing and organisational values (Hewison and Wildman, 1996).

Notwithstanding the challenges of knowledge translation, we should not dismiss theory too readily. Theories have different reach and serve different purposes. Grand theories tend to be more abstract and cover a wide terrain, whereas midrange theories are more specific and integrated in empirical reality. Unlike clinical guidelines, theories are not designed to be translated into practice in a prescriptive fashion; rather they offer frameworks for problem solving and a means for articulating decision making. Theories are also central to advancing practice and supporting knowledge sharing (Younas and Quennell, 2019). New theories are required, and established theories must evolve, to remain relevant to the dynamic nature of practice.

One reason for the invisibility of the organisational component of the nursing role is that without a language with which to describe this work, the underlying knowledge has remained largely tacit. Tacit knowledge is internalised knowledge which is acquired through experience and often referred to as the 'know how' as opposed to the 'know what' of explicit knowledge. Tacit knowledge is difficult to transfer to another person either by writing it down or verbalising it. This was pithily articulated by the polymath Michael Polanyi in the assertion, 'we can know more than we can tell' (Polanyi, 1958). Indeed, the nurses observed in *The Invisible Work of Nurses* (Allen, 2015) found it difficult to describe their practice but recognised it instantly when it was reflected to them through my observations and interpretations.

Have you ever played the game Articulate? Played in teams, the idea is to describe as many words as possible to other team members without being able to say the word itself, the length, the starting letter, any derivative or what it rhymes with or sounds like. Each turn is 30 seconds in length and the aim is to articulate as many words as possible within the available time. If you are acquainted with the game, you will be familiar with the challenges of communication where access to concepts and language is constrained. Try this with a practice example, by working through Exercise 1.1. You can record your answer in the Care Trajectory Management Workbook (see Evolve website).

EXERCISE 1.1

You are caring for a patient with renal colic, and they ask how their condition is caused. Write down how you will answer the patient's question without using any of the following words: renal, colic, kidney, urine, bladder, tissue, ureter.

Comparing the difficulties of talking about organising work with the challenges of describing practice without using certain descriptors can only be extended so far. In the earlier example, as in the game of Articulate, players still have access to a shared cultural reference for which a word exists, it is just that the rules of the game do not permit them to use it. The challenges of communication are magnified in situations of conceptual absence, as no word exists, and thus, negotiating a shared cultural reference is maximally difficult.

Ways of documenting and talking about an area of practice are central components of 'professional vision' (Goodwin, 1994). Professional vision refers to the socially organised ways of seeing and understanding events aligned with the interests or concerns of a social group. All ways of seeing are located within practice communities and reflect their specific purposes. As Goodwin (1994) illustrates, an archaeologist and a farmer will consider the same field through quite different perspectives, and each has a distinctive vocabulary for attending to and talking about features of interest. The farmer will be attuned to soil that will support varieties of crops, whereas the archaeologist will attend to stains, features and artefacts that provide evidence for earlier human activity at this location.

Nurses have conceptual resources—biological, physiological, psychological, pharmacological and sociological—with which to see and describe the patient's nursing care requirements and inform clinical decision making. No such frameworks exist for the organisational component of the nursing role. This makes it very difficult to describe nursing practice, and it constrains knowledge sharing. Gegenfurtner et al. (2019) offer a detailed analysis of how radiologists enable lay people to interpret X-ray scans. This includes using various techniques in working with the technology, but also, crucially, having terms to describe and make sense of features of the visual field, to enable the lay person to see what the expert can see. Zerubavel (1997) refers to these as practices of optical socialisation. Much of the progress in advancing practice knowledge can be attributed to the translation of tacit knowledge into explicit knowledge, which enables it to be shared (Wyatt, 2001). The concepts and theories described in this book are designed to address this gap in nursing's professional vocabulary.

Summary

This chapter has traced the history of organising work in nursing practice and has described the changes to contemporary healthcare systems that have increased the volume of activity involved in the organisation and coordination of patient care. Despite its recognised contribution to healthcare quality and safety, the organisational aspects of nursing work are not a formally acknowledged component of professional practice. For nursing to fully realise its contribution to healthcare systems, it is essential that organising work is brought out of the shadows, and the tacit knowledge that underpins it is made more explicit. Concepts and theories are an important mechanism for realising this aim.

SUMMARY OF KEY LEARNING

- Nursing work has always entailed an organisational component, and this has evolved to become a safety critical function in modern healthcare systems but is not formally recognised as such.
- The organisational components of nursing work are largely founded on tacit knowledge which makes knowledge sharing difficult.
- Concepts and theories are central to informing and advancing practice and knowledge sharing.
- Concepts enable the identification of salient features of a field of practice, talking about practice interventions and sharing practice expertise.

QUICK QUIZ

- Why has organising work had a bad press in nursing?
- What is professional vision?
- What is tacit knowledge?
- What is explicit knowledge?
- How is theory useful in nursing practice?
- What are the changes that have occurred in healthcare that have created the need for care trajectory management?

References

Allen, D., 2001. The Changing Shape of Nursing Practice: The Role of Nurses in the Hospital Division of Labour. Routledge, London and New York.

Allen, D., 2004. Re-reading nursing and re-writing practice: towards an empirically based reformulation of the nursing mandate. Nurs. Inq. 11 (4), 271–283.

Allen, D., 2015. The Invisible Work of Nurses: Hospitals, Organisation and Healthcare. Routledge, London and New York.

Allen, D., 2017. From polyformacy to formacology. BMJ Qual. Saf. 26, 695–697. doi:10.1136/bmjqs-2017-006677.

Allen, D., Purkis, M.E., Rafferty, A.M., Obstfelder, A., 2019. Integrating preparation for care trajectory management into nurse education: competencies and pedagogical strategies. Nurs. Inq. 26 (3), e12289. doi:10.1111/nin.12289.

BBC, 2013. Nurses 'drowning in a sea of paperwork'. https://www.bbc.co.uk/news/health-22206882#sans_mchannel=rss&ns_source=PublicRSS20-sa. (Accessed 12 August 2022).

Bjornsdottir, K., 2018. 'I try to make a net around each patient': home care nursing as relational practice. Scand. J. Caring Sci. 32 (1), 177–185.

Dingwall, R., 1974. Some sociological aspects of 'nursing research. Sociol. Rev. 22 (1), 45–55.

Dingwall, R., Allen, D., 2001. The implications of healthcare reforms for the profession of nursing. Nurs. Inq. 8 (2), 64–74.

Dingwall, R., Rafferty, A.M., Webster, C., 1988. An Introduction to the Social History of Nursing. Routledge, London and New York.

Exley, C., Allen, D., 2007. A critical examination of home care: end of life care as an illustrative case. Soc. Sci. Med. 65 (11), 2317–2327.

Furaker, C., 2009. Nurses' everyday activities in hospital care. J. Nurs. Manag. 17 (3), 269–277.

Garcia, R., Qureshi, I., 2022. Nurse identity: reality and media portrayal. Evid. Based Nurs. 25, 1–5.

Gegenfurtner, A., Lehtinen, E., Helle, L., Nivala, M., Svedström, E., Säljö, R., 2019. Learning to see like an expert: on the practices of professional vision and visual expertise. Int. J. Educ. Res. 98, 280–291. doi:10.1016/j.ijer.2019.09.003.

Goodwin, C., 1994. Professional vision. Am. Anthropol. 96 (3), 606–633.

Gordon, S., Nelson, S., 2006. Moving beyond the virtue script in nursing: creating a knowledge-based identity for nurses. In: Nelson, S., Gordon, S. (Eds.), The Complexities of Care: Nursing Reconsidered. Cornell University Press, Ithaca and London, pp. 13–29.

Hannigan, B., Allen, D., 2013. Complex caring trajectories in community mental health: contingencies, divisions of labor and care coordination. Commun. Ment. Health J. 49 (4), 380–388. doi:10.1007/s10597-011-9467-9.

Hayter, M., 2013. The UK Francis Report: the key messages for nursing. J. Adv. Nurs. 69 (8), e1–e3. doi:10.1111/jan.12206.

Hewison, A., Wildman, S., 1996. The theory-practice gap in nursing: a new dimension. J. Adv. Nurs. 24 (4), 754–761. doi:10.1046/j.1365-2648.1996.25214.x.

Hughes, E.C., 1984. The Sociological Eye. Transaction Books, New Brunswick and London.

Landers, M.G., 2008. The theory–practice gap in nursing: the role of the nurse teacher. J. Adv. Nurs. 32 (6), 1550–1556. doi:10.1046/j.1365-2648.2000.01605.x.

Maben, J., Latter, S., Clark, J.M., 2006. The theory-practice gap: impact of professional-bureaucratic work conflict on newly-qualified nurses. J. Adv. Nurs. 55 (4), 465–477. doi:10.1111/j.1365-2648.2006.03939.x.

Melby, L., Obstfelder, A., Hellesø, R., 2018. We tie up the loose ends': homecare nursing in a changing health care landscape. Glob. Qual. Nurs. Res. 5. doi:10.1177/2333393618816780.

Michel, L., Waelli, M., Allen, D., Minivielle, E., 2017. The content and meaning of administrative work: a qualitative study of nursing practices and perceptions. J. Adv. Nurs. 73 (9), 2179–2190. doi:10.1111/jan.13294.

Myall, M., Levett-Jones, T., Lathlean, J., 2008. Mentorship in contemporary practice: the experiences of nursing students and practice mentors. J. Clin. Nurs. 17 (14), 1834–1842. doi:10.1111/j.1365-2702.2007.02233.x.

Nelson, S., Gordon, S., 2006. Introduction. In: Nelson, S., Gordon, S. (Eds.), The Complexities of Care: Nursing Reconsidered. Cornell University Press, Ithaca and London, pp. 1–12.

Nightingale, F., 1860/1969. Notes on Nursing and Other Writings. Dover Publications Inc., New York.

Ousey, K., Gallagher, P., 2007. The theory-practice relationship in nursing: a debate. Nurse Educ. Pract. 7 (4), 199–205. doi:10.1016/j.nepr.2007.02.001.

Polanyi, M., 1958. Personal Knowledge: Towards a Post-Critical Philosophy. University of Chicago Press, Chicago.

Rolfe, G., 1993. Closing the theory-practice gap: a model of nursing praxis. J. Clin. Nurs. 2, 173–177.

Sandelowski, M., 2000. Devices & Desires: Gender, Technology and American Nursing. The University of North Carolina Press, Chapel Hill, NC.

Sharif, F., Masoumi, S., 2005. A qualitative study of nursing student experiences of clinical practice. BMC Nurs 4 (6). doi:10.1186/1472-6955-4-6.

Stephenson, J., 2018. How has nursing changed since 1948? Nurs. Times. 114 (7), 6–7.

Thorn, S., 2022. Reflections on the nursing theory movement. Nurs. Philos. doi:10.1111/nup.12406.

Timmermans, S., Berg, M., 2003. The Gold Standard: The Challenge of Evidence-Based Medicine and Standardization in Health Care. Temple University Press, Philadelphia, PA.

Wyatt, J.C., 2001. Management of explicit and tacit knowledge. J. R. Soc. Med. 94 (1), 6–9. https://journals.sagepub.com/doi/pdf/10.1177/014107680109400102.

Webb, C., 2002. Feminism, nursing and education. J. Adv. Nurs. 39 (2), 111–113.

Younas, A., Quennell, S., 2019. Usefulness of nursing theory-guided practice: an integrative review. Scand. J. Caring Sci. 33, 540–555.

Zerubavel, E., 1997. Social Mindscapes: An Invitation to Cognitive Sociology. Harvard University Press, Cambridge, MA/London, England.

Suggested Reading

Nursing Theory

Thorn, S., 2022. Reflections on the nursing theory movement. Nurs. Philos. doi:10.1111/nup.12406.
Sally Thorn offers some reflections on the history of nursing theory.

Anti-intellectualism

Hayter, M., 2013. The UK Francis Report: the key messages for nursing. J. Adv. Nurs. 69 (8), e1–e3. doi:10.1111/jan.12206.
Mark Hayter offers a perspective on how nursing is understood in the debates arising from the Francis Report, an independent public inquiry into standards of care at a UK hospital. In another example of anti-intellectualism in societal understanding of nursing work, one of the debates in the media and amongst politicians in response to the poor care exposed by Francis was how nurses are trained and, particularly, the supposed deficiencies related to graduate nurses. The argument is that nurses trained to degree level focus on theory at the expense of practical skills and lack the compassion of nurses trained through less academic or 'traditional' means.

Professional Vision

Gegenfurtner, A., Lehtinen, E., Helle, L., Nivala, M., Svedström, E., Säljö, R, 2019. Learning to see like an expert: on the practices of professional vision and visual expertise. Int. J. Educ. Res. 98, 280–291. doi:10.1016/j.ijer.2019.09.003.
A nice example of how professional vision matters for knowledge sharing.

CHAPTER 2

Care Trajectories and Care Trajectory Management

LEARNING OUTCOMES

At the end of this chapter, you will be able to:
- Understand the concepts of care trajectory and care trajectory management
- Describe how care trajectory management relates to the other components of the nursing role

Introduction

Having examined the importance of concepts for supporting professional practice and making the invisible, visible, this chapter explains and describes the two core concepts of care trajectories and care trajectory management. The aim is to introduce the ways of thinking that underpin this text and begin the process of making the connections with theoretical concepts and everyday nursing practice. Successive chapters will build on this learning to deepen your understanding of healthcare systems and nursing work; this chapter lays important foundations for the topics that follow.

From Care Pathways to Care Trajectories

In contemporary healthcare systems, it is commonplace to refer to the processes of care and treatment as a patient or clinical pathway. This metaphor has its origins in systems engineering and the aspiration that care delivery can be rationally ordered along a preplanned route. The language of a pathway is often used to communicate information to prospective patients about what to expect in their interactions with health services over the course of their care and treatment. I searched Google images using the term 'patient pathway' and found a wide assortment of diagrams depicting service processes. These ranged in style from highly formalised technical documents intended for health service managers through to patient-friendly visualisations. Despite their presentational differences, however, all had a clearly defined direction of travel at their core.

The metaphor of a pathway may have value in lessening the anxiety of prospective users by reducing the uncertainties about care and treatment. Depicting healthcare systems in this way can also be a useful mechanism through which providers involved in care delivery can comprehend complex processes (Pinder et al., 2005) and there is certainly some evidence that specific areas of healthcare can be managed effectively in this way (Allen et al., 2009; Simpson et al., 2015). But these images say little about the large volume of patients who, for a whole range of reasons, do not follow the prescribed route through the system, who, to use the vernacular, 'fall off the pathway', or who have such complex and unpredictable needs, their care and treatment could never be captured in a pathway. Thus, while healthcare systems like to behave as if processes can be managed in a linear and orderly way, it is also the case that great swathes of activity exist that defy such efforts at planning and control and must be managed more responsively. Consider the experience of Winifred Naylor (Case Study 2.1).

As Winifred's experience illustrates, healthcare has several features which create the potential for patient care to be complex and unpredictable. First, unexpected contingencies arise which

---

CASE STUDY 2.1 | **Winifred Naylor**

Winifred Naylor, an 84-year-old retired geography teacher, was admitted to hospital with a hip fracture having fallen down some steps, while tending to the garden. Prior to her accident Winfred and her husband had been living independently. They had an adult son, but the relationship had become strained in recent years and contact was infrequent.

Recovery from hip fracture varies, and to a considerable extent depends on the person's health before the accident. While in some cases hip fracture can be the result of a mechanical fall, such as a trip, it can also be a symptom of increasingly frailty, with up to 40% of people who fracture their hip having cognitive impairment (Seitz et al., 2014). The hospital responsible for Winifred's care had end-to-end patient pathways for hip fracture; these were used as rules of thumb for planning rehabilitation and discharge.

Green Pathway: This pathway was designed for patients who were fit and independent before breaking their hip, with a good level of mobility and no memory problems and needing minimal help. The pathway anticipated that patients in this category would be mobilising short distances with the physiotherapists 2 days after surgery and would be discharged within 10 days.

Amber Pathway: This pathway was designed for patients who had preexisting health conditions before breaking their hip, including mild memory problems. Patients aligned with this pathway may have needed aides to mobility before admission and may already be receiving help with domestic tasks and personal care. Patients in this group would be 'transferring out of bed' within 2 days after surgery. The indicative hospital admission would be 21 days.

Red Pathway: This pathway was designed for patients with complex health problems, limited mobility and possible memory problems. Patients in this group would already be having significant help at home or reside in supported accommodation, such as a residential of nursing home. Patients on this pathway would have a slower rehabilitation with the aim of discharging them from hospital within 28 days or slightly sooner if they were returning to supportive accommodation rather than to their own home.

As Winifred was well and living independently prior to admission, she was assigned to a Green Pathway. The expectation was that Winfred would be home within 10 days, with support from the community rehabilitation team.

The preoperative assessment concluded that Winifred was fit enough to have a general anaesthetic, and the operation took place within 24 hours of admission in alignment with clinical guidelines. The surgery and immediate postanaesthetic recovery progressed without incident. The day after the operation, Winifred was assisted to sit out of bed by the physiotherapists and was eating and drinking. She continued to make a good recovery and the team was pleased with her progress. Five days after the operation, however, Winifred experienced episodes of confusion. Although she was quite calm and lucid during the day, she became agitated and disoriented at night, expressing distrust in the motives of the nursing staff. A urine sample revealed that Winifred had an infection, for which antibiotics were prescribed. Although the delirium resolved after 3 days, Winifred felt tired and unwell and found rehabilitation exhausting. This inhibited her recovery and led to the postponement of her planned discharge. Bernard, her husband, was also very anxious about Winifred's confused state and required a lot of reassurance from staff that this was an acute episode related to the infection and not a sign of dementia, for which there was a family history.

Winifred was finally ready to return home 6 days later than planned on the Green Pathway but had to remain in hospital for an additional 3 days until the community rehabilitation team had capacity to support her at home. The ward team proposed that she could be discharged sooner with family support, but this was not acceptable to Winifred or her husband, who did not want to depend on their son. Overall, Winifred was in hospital for 19 days, moving her actual pathway closer to the 21-day Amber Pathway specified by the hospital.

stem not just from disease processes but also from a whole range of organisational and techno-logical sources. Therefore, although Winifred's surgery progressed as planned, her recovery and rehabilitation in the postoperative period were impacted by a urinary tract infection and delayed her discharge. When she was eventually ready to leave hospital, organisational issues—in the form of insufficient capacity within the community rehabilitation team—led to discharge being postponed by a further 3 days. Second, healthcare is people work, so people react to and affect the work. In the previous example, we saw how Winifred and her husband's desire to maintain their independence, and a strained relationship with their adult son, precluded the organisation of interim support at home to bridge the gap between the planned discharge date and the availability of the community rehabilitation team.

Winifred's case is not that remarkable, but it reveals how these features of healthcare work (contingency and people) create the potential for patient care to be complex and unpredictable (Strauss et al., 1985). Thus, while the metaphor of a pathway can be useful for certain purposes, it simplifies. It glosses over the unexpected infections, service constraints, changes in direction, family dynamics, differences of opinion, fears and the multiplicity of other factors that punctuate patient care and treatment. It also renders invisible the negotiations, adjustments and accommo-dations made by healthcare professionals in keeping care on track in the face of such contingen-cies. If we want to describe the organisational elements of nursing practice, we need an alternative concept that better captures the complex processes involved. This is where thinking about care *trajectories* rather than pathways has value.

The concept of a care trajectory is derived from Strauss et al.'s (1985) ideas on 'illness trajec-tories' which were set out in *Social Organisation of Medical Work*, an in-depth qualitative study of North American hospital care in the 1980s (Box 2.1). Writing in the context of a rapid growth of specialisation and bureaucratisation in health services provision, Strauss et al. argued that the term 'trajectory' was necessary to analyse the complex relationships that shape care processes.

A distinction central to the analysis [...] is that drawn between a course of illness and an illness trajectory. The first term offers no problems to the reader since everyone has experienced an illness that did not merely appear but developed gradually over time, getting worse and then perhaps clearing up. To the knowledgeable medical, nursing, and technical staffs, each kind of illness has its more or less characteristic phases, with symptoms to match, and often only skilled intervention will reverse, halt, or at least slow down the progress of the disease. Course of illness *is, then, both a common-sense and professional term.* In contrast, trajectory *is a term coined by the authors to refer not only to the physiological unfolding of a patient's disease but to the total* organization of work *done over that course, plus the* impact *on those involved with that work and its organization. For different illnesses, the trajectory will involve different medical and nursing actions, different skills and other resources, a different parcelling out of tasks among workers (including, perhaps, kin and the patient), and involving quite different relationships – instrumental and expressive both – among the workers.*

Strauss et al. (1985, p. 8, original emphasis).

BOX 2.1 ▦ Interesting Fact

Strauss was a medical sociologist, who for much of his career worked in a School of Nursing at the University of California, San Francisco. Many of his doctoral students, researchers and collaborators had nursing and/or healthcare backgrounds. Shizuko Fagerhaugh, a coauthor of *Social Organization of Medical Work*, was a sociologically trained nurse, as was Juliet Corbin, who collaborated with Strauss in studies of 'chronic illness' and developed the nursing trajectory model.

Corbin, J.M., Strauss, A., 1992. A nursing model for chronic illness management based upon the trajectory framework. In: Woog, P. (Ed.), The Chronic Illness Trajectory Framework. Springer, New York, pp. 9–28.

> **BOX 2.2 ■ Definition: Care Trajectory**
>
> 'Care trajectory' refers to 'the unfolding of a patient's health and social care needs, the total organisation of work carried out over its course, and the impact on those involved with that work and its organisation'.
>
> _____
>
> With permission from Allen, D., Griffiths, L., Lyne, P., 2004. Understanding complex trajectories in health and social care provision. Sociol. Health Illn. 26(7), 1008–1030.

For Strauss et al., the illness trajectory concept is a means for identifying and understanding the immense variety of events that occur as patients, kin and staff seek to control and cope with illnesses. They describe in detail the evolution of individual illness trajectories observed during the study, documenting the resources and types of work involved, and the complex clinical, organisational and psychosocial issues that shape patient care and treatment. While the technical details may be a little dated now, these descriptions offer a window into real-life processes not captured by the formal organisational plan or pathway diagrams and which bring into view the matters of concern that form the substance of nurses' organising work.

But Strauss et al. did not explicitly study nurses' work. In fact, their analysis deliberately focused on categories of *work* rather than the *workers*. In building on these ideas for the purposes of describing and explaining nursing practice, I have replaced the concept of illness trajectory with the concept of a care trajectory (Box 2.2). This shift in language reflects several considerations. First, *Social Organisation of Medical Work* was a hospital-based study, and the analysis is implicitly founded on a medical model. It did not include trajectories which involved progression from the acute sector to community and social care. By reframing the concept using the language of care, rather than illness, attention is focused on the activity involved in the care of the person rather than the sickness (Allen et al., 2004). Second, in studies that have built on Strauss et al.'s work, the emphasis on illness has created a tendency to focus on individual experiences of disease processes, rather than deepening understanding of the systems of care which give rise to these experiences, and it is the latter that I wish to foreground for the purposes of understanding the organisational components of nursing work. By shifting the language from illness to care, experiences of illness are decentred, and the focus remains on patient needs, *and* the work associated with meeting those needs *and* the impact on those involved. It is these relationships that are at the heart of the organisational component of the nursing role.

From Care Trajectories to Care Trajectory Management

Having made the case for incorporating the language of care trajectories in nursing's professional vocabulary, the next logical step is to embrace the concept of care trajectory *management*. Care trajectory management is the overarching term developed for describing the organisational component of the nursing role, which has hitherto had no name (Allen, 2018). If we think about a care trajectory as the network of elements involved in a patient's care—people; departments and organisations; materials, equipment and technologies; knowledge and information; and activities—then care trajectory *management* refers to the role of nurses in mobilising, coordinating and organising these relationships, to hold together patient care. Consider the following vignette:

> It is 1130 and Maureen has paused at the Nurses' Station to review progress. The ward is the calmest it's been all day. Only a few individuals have yet to be washed and everyone scheduled for theatre this afternoon is prepared. Sunlight has started to flood into the corridor from the ward areas as one by one the curtains that have enfolded the bed spaces since shortly after breakfast are drawn back. Maureen has just completed processing a newly admitted patient and inserts the various

assessment tools, care plans and record forms into the patient's file. She places the medication chart prominently on the Nurses' Station and affixes to it a note requesting that the doctor prescribe night sedation which, she has established, the patient usually takes to help her sleep. Maureen removes a sheet of paper from her pocket, unfolds it and scrutinises the content. It is a list of all patients on the unit; for each a complex set of symbols denotes the current status of their care. Some of these inscriptions are in blue, some in red. The latter is information Maureen has added having attended the ward round earlier. It is her practice to colour code her entries so she can identify readily new developments to be passed on to the person responsible. Several issues now have been attended to: the junior doctor has prescribed medication for the patients going home tomorrow; the discharge letters for the community nursing service are prepared; and the receptionist has been instructed to arrange out-patient appointments. Maureen ticks off these items on her sheet and glances at the clock. There is just enough time to telephone the social worker to check the progress of Mr White's home care arrangements before she must leave for the morning meeting to discuss the bed state. All today's discharges are going ahead, but she knows the elective admissions are likely to remain on hold as there are patients in the Emergency Unit who require beds. She hopes she will not have to accept patients for whom another service is responsible as the work of organising care for 'outliers' is more difficult but recognises this is sometimes necessary. Maureen picks up the telephone but quickly returns it to the receiver when she notices that the colorectal nurse specialist has arrived on the unit. She knows she will want an update on Mrs Banner. As they are talking, Maureen takes the opportunity to ask about another patient whose stoma management is interfering with their wound care. The colorectal nurse agrees to change the appliance. Maureen makes a note to this effect on her list. She is now running late for the meeting, so she quickly surveys the bed board and heads off down the corridor. En route she encounters a rather lost-looking junior doctor who inquires, 'Where do you keep purple blood bottles?' 'In there' Maureen replies, pointing to a cupboard on her right and, without breaking her stride, she disappears out of the ward.

(With permission from Taylor & Francis Group. Allen, D., 2015. The Invisible Work of Nurses: Hospitals, Organisation and Healthcare. Routledge, London and New York, pp. 1–2.)

This example offers a momentary glimpse into the working life of a hospital nurse. Despite the absence of crisis, drama or heroic interventions, it captures much of the critical work nurses do to ensure the quality and safety of patient care: work to maintain an overview of patients' care, work to manage information flows, work to ensure that all essential activities are carried out and do not interfere with each other, work in assembling the materials and resources required and work to support the transfer of patients across the healthcare system. The example also illustrates a distinctive professional 'habitus' (Bourdieu, 1980): a way of *seeing* healthcare that entails zooming in and attending to individual patients, and zooming out to review the wider clinical environment; a way of *understanding* healthcare, which involves a synthesis of clinical and organisational knowledge; and a way of *acting* in healthcare which entails standing between the different parts of the system and doing what is necessary to connect them together (Box 2.3). This is the work of care trajectory management, and yet while a highly skilled nursing function, it has hitherto had no name.

BOX 2.3 ■ Definition: Habitus

The concept of habitus was developed by the French sociologist Bourdieu (1980). Habitus refers to socially acquired habits, skills and dispositions, which shape how individuals perceive the social world around them and react to it. Habitus evolves over time as individuals navigate the social world. Habitus is neither a result of free will nor determined by structures, but created by a kind of interplay between the two over time. People with similar backgrounds and opportunities develop a shared habitus.

Bourdieu, P., 1980. The Logic of Practice. Stanford University Press, Stanford.

Care Trajectory Management and the Nursing Role

Care trajectory management has a synergistic relationship with the other dimensions of the nursing role. It overlaps with but is distinct from direct clinical care, and unit management. Whereas the former is patient focused, and the latter is focused on the environment for care, care trajectory management is trajectory focused. While it is possible to think about patient care activities and management of the care environment as distinct domains of work, care trajectory management is not a discrete activity. It is a way of perceiving, understanding and acting that is woven through the fabric of everyday nursing practice and interleaved with clinical and unit management work. Founded on the integration of clinical and organisational knowledge, care trajectory management is a responsive practice which requires oversight of emergent processes, flexible decision making and creative reactions to the evolution of trajectories. It entails standing between the different parts of the system and doing what is necessary to connect them together, whether this is progressing scheduled plans, or recognising and reacting to unexpected developments, such as changing patient needs and shifts in the care environment. This is highly skilled work, which depends on a distinctive professional vision, and the ability to manage complex care processes, in turbulent environments (Allen et al., 2019).

Summary

This chapter has introduced the core concepts of the text—care trajectory and care trajectory management—and has explained the intellectual heritage of these ideas and the rationale for their selection to describe the organisational aspects of nursing work. The relationship of care trajectory management with the wider nursing role, and the distinctive way of seeing, understanding and acting in healthcare that characterises this component of nursing practice have been described. Subsequent chapters build on these concepts. First, it is important to examine more closely those features of healthcare work that make care trajectory management necessary.

SUMMARY OF KEY LEARNING

- The concepts of care trajectory and care trajectory management have been adopted to describe the organisational components of nursing practice because they accommodate the complexity and unpredictable qualities of the organisation of patient care and treatment.

QUICK QUIZ

- Why is *care trajectory* a preferrable term to *patient pathway*?
- What elements are included in the concept of a care trajectory?
- Which elements of nursing practice does care trajectory management refer to?

References

Allen, D., 2015. The Invisible Work of Nurses: Hospitals, Organisation and Healthcare. Routledge, London and New York.

Allen, D., 2018. Care trajectory management: a conceptual framework for formalising emergent organisation in nursing practice. J. Nurs. Manag. 27 (1), 4–9.

Allen, D., Gillen, E., Rixson, L., 2009. A systematic review of the effectiveness of integrated care pathways: what works, for whom, in which circumstances? Int. J. Evid. Based Healthcare. 7, 61–74.

Allen, D., Griffiths, L., Lyne, P., 2004. Understanding complex trajectories in health and social care provision. Sociol. Health Illn. 26 (7), 1008–1030.

Allen, D., Purkis, M.E., Rafferty, A.M., Obstfelder, A., 2019. Integrating preparation for care trajectory management into nurse education: competencies and pedagogical strategies. Nurs. Inq 26 (3), e12289. doi:10.1111/nin.12289.

Bourdieu, P., 1980. The Logic of Practice. Stanford University Press, Stanford.

Pinder, R., Petchey, R., Shaw, S., Carter, Y., 2005. What's in a care pathway? Towards a cultural cartography of the new NHS. Sociol. Health Illn 27 (6), 759–779.

Seitz, D.P., Gill, S.S., Gruneir, A., Austin, P.C., Anderson, G.M., Bell, C.M., et al., 2014. Effects of dementia on postoperative outcomes of older adults with hip fractures: a population-based study. J. Am. Med. Dir. Assoc. 15 (5), 334–341.

Simpson, J.C., Moonesinghe, S.R., Grocott, M.P.W., Kuper, M., McMeeking, A., Oliver, C.M., et al., 2015. Enhanced recovery from surgery in the UK: an audit of the enhanced recovery partnership programme 2009–2012. Br. J. Anaesth. 115 (4), 560–568.

Strauss, A., Fagerhaugh, S., Suczet, B., Wiener, C., 1985. Social Organization of Medical Work. University of Chicago Press, Chicago, IL.

Suggested Reading

Patient Pathways

Pinder, R., Petchey, R., Shaw, S., Carter, Y., 2005. What's in a care pathway? Towards a cultural cartography of the new NHS. Sociol. Health Illn. 27 (6), 759–779. doi:10.1111/j.1467-9566.2005.00473.x.

A rare insight into the processes of pathway construction, which reveals the different perspectives of participants in service processes and makes it abundantly clear that these practices as far from objective and value free. What maps silence is as interesting as what they make visible, and we should guard against mistaking the map for the territory.

Care Trajectory Management and the Wider Nursing Role

Jackson, J., Anderson, J.E., Maben, J., 2021. What is nursing work? A meta-narrative review and integrated framework. Int. J. Nurs. Stud. 122, 103944. doi:10.1016/j.ijnurstu.2021.103944.

An ambitious paper, which reviews the research evidence on nursing work, including care trajectory management.

The Complexities of Healthcare Work

LEARNING OUTCOMES

At the end of this chapter, you will be able to:
- Outline the seven complexities of healthcare work that make its organisation difficult
- Identify the potential sources of complexity in trajectories of care
- Describe the properties of complex adaptive systems

Introduction

This chapter explores in detail those features of healthcare work that contribute to the unpredictability of trajectories of care. When I was writing about my research findings on the invisible work of nurses, I realised that to really understand the organisational component of the nursing role and see nursing differently, it was necessary to understand and see healthcare systems differently too. Studying the everyday practices of nurses highlighted what healthcare systems look like from within rather than how they are depicted in formal organisational plans, pathways or patient information leaflets. My analysis revealed that for much of the time, an individual's trajectory of care is an amorphous network of diverse elements—symptoms, signs, assessments, test results, treatment regimes, specialist knowledge, emotions, providers, technologies, plans—which evolves dynamically in response to changes in disease processes, decisions around care and treatment, and shifts in the wider care environment. It is through the work that nurses do in making sense of these relationships and integrating the different moving parts that patient care is organised, order is created and concerted action is enabled.

In the practice setting, nurses, like other healthcare professionals, experience this complexity every day (Box 3.1). It takes time to develop the skills required to make sense of and respond to

---

BOX 3.1 ■ The Turbulent Environment of Hospital Nursing

In a classic sociological study of nursing work, Melia (1979) draws an analogy between the organisation of work in the coal-mining industry and the work of hospital ward nurses. She draws on empirical data generated in an observational study carried out in 50 hospital wards (Moult et al., 1978) and deploys systems thinking in her analysis. A central concern in systems thinking is the interaction between the production process and the work environment. In nursing, the production process is the care of patients, and the environment is the ward or clinical context in which that care takes place.

Emery and Trist (1965) applied systems thinking to the coal-mining industry and classified the production environments according to their complexity. The classification ranged from a placid environment to that of a 'turbulent field'. A turbulent field is an environment that is unstable and liable to disorganisation and so demands a particular form of work organisation for production to continue. Emery and Trist argue that work undertaken in turbulent fields can be analysed in terms of its two key components: the primary task and the skills and mechanisms involved in coping with the work environment. Drawing on this work, Melia argues that the turbulent environment of the coalface is comparable with the work environment of the ward. Therefore, simply counting the tasks involved in patient care misses many of the activities and skills involved in nursing work.

Emery, F.E., Trist, E.L., 1965. The causal texture of organizational environments. Hum. Relat. 18 (i), 21–31.

Melia, K.M., 1979. A sociological approach to the analysis of nursing work. J. Adv. Nurs. 4, 57–67.

Moult, A., Hockey, L., Melia, K.M., 1978. Unpublished report for the Leverhulme Trustees.

EXERCISE 3.1

Reflection

Before reading further, take some time to reflect on your first experience of a healthcare setting as a student. Where was it? What features of the environment most readily spring to mind? How did you feel? Really immerse yourself in that moment. You can record your answer in the Care Trajectory Management Workbook so that you can refer to it as your learning progresses (see Evolve website).

---

the turbulence of the healthcare work environment, and to develop the habitus (Bourdieu, 1980) described in Chapter 2 (see Care Trajectories and Care Trajectory Management) (Benner, 1984; Benner and Tanner, 1987; Hansten and Washburn, 2000). For some, including my 19-year-old self, this disorder can be overwhelming (Allen, 2015; Melia, 1979). Understanding the sources of this complexity is, then, a key pillar of the care trajectory management knowledge base (Exercise 3.1).

The Seven Complexities of Healthcare Work

In previous chapters I have argued that the need for care trajectory management arises from the complexity of healthcare work, which produces unstable trajectories of care and unstable work environments. But what are the causes of this complexity? This section delves deeper into the anatomy and physiology of healthcare systems to examine seven sources of complexity. Each complexity has a complementary exercise designed to support the application of these insights to practice. The exercises in this section (Exercises 3.2–3.8) are based on Case Study 3.1. You can record your answers in the Care Trajectory Management Workbook (see Evolve website).

COMPLEXITY 1: HEALTHCARE IS A WORK OF MANY HANDS

Healthcare is a work of 'many hands' (Aveling et al., 2016). Over the last century there has been an explosion of roles, professions and specialisms in healthcare, and the workforce continues to evolve

CASE STUDY 3.1	Gareth Williams

Gareth Williams is a 54-year-old production manager in the South Wales steel industry. He lives with his wife Meryl in a home that they own, which overlooks the ocean. The couple enjoy a daily walk along the coastal path with their dog, Troy.

Gareth is a member of a local football club, a group of enthusiastic amateurs, which meets once a week for a friendly game followed by a postmatch debrief in the local 'pub'. Gareth smokes 10 cigarettes a day, having cut back on a 40-a-day habit in the last year. Despite remaining active, he has gained weight, with his wife describing him as 'cuddly'.

On Wednesday evening Gareth decided not to go to football and went to bed early complaining of feeling unwell. On waking the next morning, Gareth was confused, one side of his face had dropped, and he had a weakness in his arm and leg. He had also been incontinent of urine.

Meryl immediately recognised the signs of a stroke and called the emergency medical services. An ambulance arrived swiftly—stroke is a recognised priority call—and Gareth was taken directly to the university teaching hospital, a designated stroke thrombolysis centre. The ambulance crew had given the department advanced warning of their arrival and an urgent computerised tomography (CT) scan had been arranged. Gareth was taken directly to the CT scan which determined that the cause of the stroke was a clot and Gareth was deemed to be a candidate for thrombolysis—clot busting therapy.

As the intervention is time-critical, the thrombolysis team was quickly mobilised, with all the materials required for the procedure having been organised in advance by the specialist nurse stroke coordinator. Following the procedure, Gareth was monitored in the department, and then transferred to the acute stroke unit.

Initial assessment by the medical team revealed that Gareth had no communication or cognitive problems, but some residual weaknesses in his right arm and leg. He also experienced some swallowing difficulties. A routine urine test revealed high blood glucose levels, and following blood tests, Gareth was diagnosed with type 2 diabetes. This was considered mild, and manageable through medication, weight loss and adjustments to diet.

Gareth made a very good recovery. His swallowing difficulties resolved within a week, and he regained the use of his arm and leg, although sometimes struggled with balance and coordination. Gareth threw himself into rehabilitation with enthusiasm, determined to return to his previous levels of fitness and eager to get home. He felt isolated in the hospital. While he appreciated the privacy of having a single-occupancy room, after the first few days, he saw little of the nurses, and his primary recurring social contacts were with catering and domestic staff, and his daily rehabilitation with the physiotherapist.

Gareth was discharged from hospital into the care of the community healthcare team; he was prescribed nicotine patches, aspirin, metformin (for his diabetes) and medication for constipation. The physiotherapist provided him with a patient information leaflet with instructions for exercises at home; the dietician provided written advice on diet. The occupational therapist offered to fit handrails in the bathroom and along the set of steps to the house, but Gareth refused; he felt he could manage, and he was concerned that Meryl, who was very house proud, would not welcome these modifications to their home. The couple also declined the support of the community resource team; Meryl felt she was able to support Gareth's recovery and the hospital team concluded that she would be able to manage. The final preparations for discharge were coordinated by the ward nurses, who ensured that everything required was in place on the day of discharge: medications to take home, information leaflets, a letter for the primary care doctor.

After the initial euphoria of returning home, Gareth experienced extreme fatigue. He became depressed, as he tried to process what had happened to him, and its impact on his self-identity. Although his friends from football offered to take him to the pub, Gareth refused. He felt diminished by the stroke. Meryl, who had always taken responsibility for food preparation, embraced fully the dietary guidance provided by the hospital dietician. But Gareth took little pleasure in his meals and ate little; he also complained about a metallic taste in his mouth. To encourage Gareth to eat and elevate his mood, after a few weeks, Meryl reverted to the meals and snacks Gareth had previously enjoyed. Although this had a positive impact on Gareth's enthusiasm for food and his energy levels, Meryl worried about its effects on Gareth's diabetes management. She sought advice from the primary care practice nurse and was reassured that in the short-term, a flexible approach was acceptable, given Gareth's mental health.

While Gareth's appetite improved, he lacked the motivation to carry out the recommended exercises for his rehabilitation and complained that he could not understand the exercise information leaflet provided by the hospital physiotherapist. His progress stalled. Concerned about the impact of Gareth's mental health on his recovery, Meryl persuaded him to see his primary care doctor, who agreed to refer

Continued

CASE STUDY 3.1	Gareth Williams—cont'd

him for community physiotherapy but warned that there was a waiting list. He also made a referral to a stroke support group.

Gareth did not want his condition to define him and initially attended the stroke support group with reluctance. Despite his early reservations, this proved to be a significant source of social solidarity and advice and he continued to attend regularly. It also prompted him to pay privately for physiotherapy rather than waiting for the hospital referral, a strategy recommended by members of the group.

After 6 months Gareth's mental health improved, he was starting to do more and had visited the pub to see his friends from the football group and had resumed dog walking. Just as he was considering a phased return to work, he suffered a hypoglycaemic episode while out walking. Frightened by the event, he made an appointment to see his primary care doctor who referred him to the community dietician for advice on managing his diet as his activity levels increased and reinforced the importance of losing weight. His rehabilitation continued to progress, and Gareth hoped to be able to return to playing football.

in response to new technologies, scientific advances and demographic and organisational changes. Beyond nursing and midwifery, at the time of writing, the UK National Health Service (NHS) website boasted 350 careers, including allied health professions, ambulance services, healthcare scientists, technicians, medical associates, therapists, pharmacists, social workers, support roles and 24 medical specialities (https://www.healthcareers.nhs.uk/explore-roles). Many of the individuals involved in a trajectory may never meet the patient but act at a distance to influence care and treatment: they examine bodily tissues and blood results, they dispense medications, they interpret scans and X-rays, they develop prostheses, they prepare specialist diets.

As well as being a work of many hands, the collective endeavour of healthcare work typically spans multiple departments and organisations, each with distinctive functions, organisation and governance structures, working practices, referral criteria and funding mechanisms. Even in simple cases, a patient's care typically extends across different teams and organisations, and trajectories frequently entail transitions between different services.

Healthcare work is not confined to formal occupations, and professions, of course. The increasing prevalence of long-term conditions requires patients to engage in a multiplicity of everyday management practices—self-monitoring, controlling diet, medication regimes—and the range of tasks expands significantly in cases of multimorbidity (May et al., 2014) (Box 3.2). It is also the case that family members and significant others provide substantial sources of support—direct care, surveillance and coordination (Allen, 2000; Corbin and Strauss, 1988). Indeed, many community care arrangements are possible only by dint of the work of family and or significant others (Hannigan and Allen, 2013). So, understanding healthcare as a work of many hands should not be restricted to the hands of healthcare professionals alone. Bear this in mind, as you work through Exercise 3.2.

BOX 3.2 ■ Burden of Treatment Theory

May et al. (2014) developed 'burden of treatment theory' to conceptualise the growing volume and complexity of healthcare work required of individuals and their social networks in the management of long-term conditions. An important impetus for the theory was to reframe debates in healthcare practices about nonadherence to treatment regimens to focus on the resources individuals require to achieve these ends.

May, C.R., Eton, D.T., Boehmer, K., Gallacher, K., Hunt, K., MacDonald, S., et al., 2014. Rethinking the patient: using Burden of Treatment Theory to understand the changing dynamics of illness. BMC Health Serv. Res. 14(281). doi:10.1186/1472-6963-14-281.

EXERCISE 3.2

List all the people, departments or services involved in Gareth William's acute care from the onset of the stroke to his discharge home. Don't worry if you do not know all the precise role titles.

You can record your answer in the Care Trajectory Management Workbook (see Evolve website).

COMPLEXITY 2: HEALTHCARE IS TECHNOLOGICALLY RICH

Healthcare involves a wide array of technologies. Nurses work with a variety of tools, instruments and machines to care for patients, even if they have not always thought of these devices as technologies (Sandelowski, 2000). In everyday use the term 'technology' tends to be reserved for sophisticated equipment, but research on healthcare technologies typically takes a broader view (Heath et al., 2003; Timmermans and Berg, 2003) which is how we will be thinking about technologies throughout this text. Framed in this way, in understanding the technological richness of healthcare, it is important to look beyond the immediately obvious examples such as complex surgical and diagnostic devices and extend our focus to include pharmacological technologies (medications, infusions, wound dressings) (Prout, 1996), information technologies (databases, computers, telephones) (Berg, 1997; Dent, 1990) and the mundane technologies of everyday care such as beds, charts, white boards, pens and paper (Allen 2016; Hardey et al., 2000; Heath 1982).

Beyond the role of technology in healthcare practice, people depend on an array of technologies to live their daily 'autonomous' lives. These so-called assistive technologies include hearing devices, spectacles, walking aides, wheelchairs, communication aides, pill organisers and safety alarms (Winance, 2006). Globally, more than 1 billion people need one or more assistive technology. With an ageing population, more than 2 billion people will require one assistive technology by 2030, with many older people needing two or more. Assistive technology reduces the need for formal health and support services, long-term care and the work of caregivers. Without assistive technology, people are often excluded, isolated and locked into poverty, thereby increasing the impact of disease and disability on a person, their family and society (WHO, 2018).

As technologies change, so does healthcare. New technologies revolutionise patient diagnosis, care and treatment; they can also transform the organisation and management of healthcare systems and reshape professional practice (Box 3.3). The comparative stagnation of nursing in the 1950s, for example, was at least partly the result of the antibiotic revolution in medicine. Many of the core skills of nursing patients with fevers and sepsis were wiped out almost overnight (Dingwall and Allen, 2001). Advances in pharmacology were a factor in the transformation and deinstitutionalisation of mental

---

BOX 3.3 ■ Transformational Therapy Cures Haemophilia B

On 21 July 2022, James Gallagher, the BBC health and science correspondent, reported on the results of a trial of a new therapy to correct a genetic defect that causes haemophilia B.

Haemophilia B is a condition caused by insufficient clotting factor IX. People with the condition must take injections of factor IX to prevent serious bleeding; many restrict their everyday activities to manage the risk of injury, and many experience complications—for example, debilitating joint pain—because of the condition.

At the time of the report, it was predicted that most adults with haemophilia B would be cured in 3 years. Underlining the transformational impacts of new technologies, Professor Pratima Chowdary, a specialist consultant from the Royal Free Hospital and University College London, who was involved in the trial, told the journalist that she's now 'looking for my next job' as curing haemophilia 'will be a reality for the majority of adults in the next one to three years' (Gallagher, 2022).

Gallagher, J., 2022. Transformational therapy cures haemophilia B. https://www.bbc.co.uk/news/health-62240061 (Accessed 30 November 2022).

EXERCISE 3.3

List all the technologies involved in Gareth's care in hospital and at home. Let your imagination roam freely; don't just focus on sophisticated equipment, consider everyday technologies too. What functions do these technologies perform? How do these technologies impact on Gareth Williams' care?

You can record your answer in the Care Trajectory Management Workbook (see Evolve website).

health services, witnessed over the last 30 years (The Health Foundation and The King's Fund, 2015). Healthcare systems across the world have been impacted significantly by the COVID-19 pandemic. New vaccines have been developed and administered at pace; preexisting technologies have been deployed to facilitate healthcare provision in COVID-secure ways, and programmes of research and development have been rapidly mobilised to address the new health and societal challenges created by the pandemic. The legacy effects of these innovations on healthcare practice and the wider society are likely to be profound. Return to Case Study 3.1 and work through Exercise 3.3.

COMPLEXITY 3: HEALTHCARE IS DISTRIBUTED WORK

There is a lot of talk about 'teamwork' in healthcare, but for much of the time, activity is widely distributed in time and space with providers making largely independent contributions to patient care and treatment. Each member of the healthcare team operates with a singular understanding of the patient reflecting their individual work purposes.

There is, quite literally, no single individual who possesses complete knowledge about any given patient.

Ellingsen and Monteiro (2003, p. 204)

The work practices that characterise trajectories of care are an example of distributed cognition (Hutchins, 1995). This term is used to describe situations in which knowledge is dispersed over a community of individuals and external artefacts, rather than being represented in individual brains (Box 3.4).

It is not uncommon in collaborative work situations for participants to vary in the knowledge they possess, and research in this field attends to the arrangements that need to be in place to enable them to pool resources, align their efforts and negotiate to accomplish tasks. Healthcare systems are punctuated by a whole host of coordination mechanisms designed for this purpose (Schmidt and Simone, 1996). These include formal events such as handovers or hand-offs, ward rounds, case conferences and multidisciplinary meetings, as well as devices such as white boards, ICT (information and communication technology) systems and patient records and informal processes developed by frontline staff (Box 3.5 for some critical insights). Use these insights to reflect on Case Study 3.1 (Exercise 3.4).

BOX 3.4 ■ Distributed Cognition

Hutchins (1995) applied the distributed cognition approach to the analysis of cockpits in commercial airlines to show how the cockpit system—rather than the pilot and copilot—performs the tasks of counting and remembering a set of correspondences between airspeed and wing configuration.

It is not the cognitive performance and expertise of any one single person or machine that are important for the continued operation or the landing and take-off of airplanes. The cognition is distributed over the personnel, sensors and machinery both in the plane and on the ground, including but not limited to the controllers, pilots and the crew.

Hutchins, E., 1995. How a cockpit remembers its speeds. Cogn. Sci. 19, 265–288.

> **BOX 3.5 ■ Insights From Distributed Cognition on Healthcare Information Systems**
>
> Hazlehurst et al. (2008) argue that much of the dissatisfaction of medical information systems is the failure of developers to appreciate the distributed character of healthcare work. They argue that medical informatics has been guided by an individual-centred model of human cognition, in which knowledge, problem solving and information processing are understood as performed by the minds of an individual agent or healthcare professional. This helps to explain why many cutting-edge information technologies have not been normalised in practice, have created challenges for users, produce significant workflow challenges and adverse safety impacts.
>
> Hazlehurst, B., Gorman, P.N., McMullena, C.K., 2008. Distributed cognition: an alternative model of cognition for medical informatics. Int. J. Med. Inform. 77, 226–234.

EXERCISE 3.4

It is 4 days after Gareth Williams was admitted to hospital with an acute stroke. His care and progress will be reviewed at the ward round. Return to the list you generated in Exercise 3.1 and identify which actors are currently involved in Gareth's care. For each actor identified, write down which aspects of Gareth's care they are knowledgeable about. Now reflect on your experiences of a typical ward round and consider who, from your list, is likely to be present for the event? How is the knowledge of absent participants built into discussions and decision making?

You can record your answer in the Care Trajectory Management Workbook (see Evolve website).

COMPLEXITY 4: ILLNESS AND RECOVERY ARE UNPREDICTABLE

Illness and recovery processes are not predictable, which makes trajectory management challenging. Much of healthcare work is nonroutine, so it is difficult to preschedule events and activities. It is also the case that with an ageing population, many patients have additional health conditions and social factors that increase the complexity of therapeutic management and impact on treatment and recovery. For example, patients with preexisting dementia have a greater than average risk of early death after surgery, and their incidence of fatal complications is higher than that of surgical patients without dementia (Kassahun, 2018); people with diabetes have higher risks of infectious complications and in-hospital mortality following surgery than patients without diabetes (Lin et al., 2019); and people with a long-term physical condition are more than twice as likely to develop mental ill health (Mental Health Foundation, 2022).

Shippee et al. (2012) developed a 'cumulative complexity model' to illustrate how clinical and social factors amass and interact to complicate patient care. Patient complexity is understood as a dynamic status which accumulates over time, with individual factors interacting with each other in emergent ways. For example, mental health problems can make it harder for people to cope with a physical health condition (Mental Health Foundation, 2022); mobility problems can make it more difficult to undertake cardiac rehabilitation; and we know that people with preexisting health conditions are more severely impacted by COVID-19. The use of multiple medicines, commonly referred to as polypharmacy, is also increasingly common (Box 3.6). Complete Exercise 3.5 to apply these insights to Case Study 3.1.

EXERCISE 3.5

Return to Case Study 3.1 and identify any aspects of Gareth's illness and recovery that made, or had the potential to make, his trajectory of care unpredictable?

You can record your answer in the Care Trajectory Management Workbook (see Evolve website).

BOX 3.6 ■ Polypharmacy

Polypharmacy is associated with adverse outcomes including mortality, falls, adverse drug reactions, increased length of stay in hospital and readmission to hospital soon after discharge (Caughey et al., 2010, cited by Masnoon et al., 2017; Milton et al., 2008). The risk of adverse outcomes grows with increasing numbers of medications (Maher et al., 2014, cited by Masnoon et al., 2017), and can result from a multitude of factors including the interactions of medications and the interaction of medications with disease processes. Older patients are at even greater risk of adverse effects because of decreased renal and hepatic function, lower lean body mass and reduced hearing, vision, cognition and mobility (Bushardt et al., 2008, cited by Masnoon et al., 2017).

Bushardt, R.L., Massey, E.B., Simpson, T.W., Ariail, J.C., Simpson, K.N., 2008. Polypharmacy: misleading, but manageable. Clin. Interv. Aging. 3(2), 383–389. doi:10.2147/CIA.S2468.

Caughey, G.E., Roughead, E.E., Pratt, N., Shakib, S., Vitry, A.I., Gilbert, A.L., 2010. Increased risk of hip fracture in the elderly associated with prochlorperazine: is a prescribing cascade contributing? Pharmacoepidemiol. Drug Saf. 19(9), 977–982. doi:10.1002/pds.2009.

Maher, R.L., Hanlon, J., Hajjar, E.R., 2014. Clinical consequences of polypharmacy in elderly. Exp. Opin. Drug Saf. 3(1), 57–65. doi:10.1517/14740338.2013.827660.

Masnoon, N., Shakib, S., Kalisch-Ellett, L., Caughey, G.E., 2017. What is polypharmacy? A systematic review of definitions. BMC Geriatr. 17(1), 230. doi:10.1186/s12877-017-0621-2.

Milton, J.C., Hill-Smith, I., Jackson, S.H.D., 2008. Prescribing for older people. Br. Med. J. 336(7644), 606–609. doi:10.1136/bmj.39503.424653.80.

COMPLEXITY 5: HEALTHCARE IS PEOPLE WORK

Healthcare is people work. Patients have a stake in their care and treatment and so do their family and significant others. Whereas historically, healthcare was organised according to a model of medical dominance in which healthcare providers knew best and patients were required to follow professional advice, in contemporary healthcare systems, there is a growing emphasis on patient-centred care, shared decision making and family involvement. Even though research suggests that the asymmetries of power that characterised traditional models of practice are remarkably persistent across all healthcare professions (Allen, 2000; Pilnick and Dingwall, 2011), and often with good reason (Pilnick, 2022), it is nevertheless the case that patients and families have a view on their care and treatment, and this impacts on healthcare organisation.

I was a member of a team of researchers who carried out a study of interprofessional working at the health and social care interface in patients who had suffered a first acute stroke (Allen et al., 2000). In-depth qualitative case studies, using a combination of observations and interviews, were undertaken of eight individual's care trajectories in two different health regions over 6 months as they progressed from acute to community care.

Stroke causes 'biographical disruption' (Bury, 1982), changing one's sense of self and identity (Box 3.7). The research highlighted how following a stroke, patients and families needed time to adjust to their altered circumstances and make the necessary modifications to their lives, but this conflicted with the pressures to discharge patients from hospital experienced by health and social care staff. For example, Rosa Jackson's discharge was delayed because of a disagreement between health and social services staff and the family about the appropriate discharge destination. Health and social services staff favoured a nursing home placement because of Rosa's dependency: she was doubly incontinent and immobile and required pressure area care. However, her daughter and granddaughter strongly resisted the idea. They were a close family and prior to her discharge had provided considerable support for Rosa. Despite the efforts of service providers to persuade the family that a nursing home was the 'best' discharge

BOX 3.7 ■ Biographical Disruption

Bury (1982) developed the concept of 'biographical disruption' to refer to how a life-changing illness interferes with an individual's social or cultural experiences by threatening self-identity. Bury's original work examined the onset and diagnosis of rheumatoid arthritis. The participants in his study experienced ruptures in the 'taken for granted assumptions and behaviours' that structured their daily lives (Bury, 1982, p. 169).

Many studies have subsequently used the concept of biographical disruption to better understand how individuals are impacted by injury and illness and how identity is managed in the face of these effects. Engman (2019) offers a very useful overview of the applications of the theory which include motor neuron disease (Locock et al., 2009), Crohn's disease (Saunders, 2017), stroke (Faircloth et al., 2004), fibromyalgia (Asbring, 2001), HIV (Carricaburu and Peirret, 1995), mental illness (Apesoa-Varano et al., 2015; Perry and Pescsolodio, 2012) and breast cancer (Liamputtong and Suwankhong, 2015).

While many studies, following Bury, have highlighted the disruptive impacts of illness on identity and sense of self, others have also shown how people are able to normalise the condition over time (Bell et al., 2016; Sanderson et al., 2011). The supplementary concept of biographic flows has also been introduced to identify the impact of an individual's diagnosis on the wider family (Castellanos et al., 2018).

Apesoa-Varano, E.C., Barker, J.C., Hinton, L., 2015. Shards of sorrow: older men's accounts of their depression experience. Soc. Sci. Med. 124, 1–8.

Asbring, P., 2001. Chronic illness – a disruption in life: identity-transformation among women with chronic fatigue syndrome and fibromyalgia. J. Adv. Nurs. 34(3), 312–319.

Bell, S.L., Tyrrell, J., Phoenix, C., 2016. Ménière's disease and biographical disruption: where family transitions collide. Soc. Sci. Med. 166, 177–185. doi:10.1016/j.socscimed.2016.08.025.

Bury, M., 1982. Chronic illness as biographical disruption. Sociol. Health Illn. 4(2), 167–182.

Carricaburu, D., Pierret, J., 1995. From biographical disruption to biographical reinforcement: the case of HIV-positive men. Sociol. Health Illn. 17(1), 65–88.

Castellanos, M.E.P., Barros, N.F., Coelho, S.S., 2018. Biographical ruptures and flows in the family experience and trajectory of children with cystic fibrosis. Cien Saude Colet. 23(2), 357–368. Portuguese, English. doi:10.1590/1413-81232018232.16252017.

Engman, A., 2019. Embodiment and the foundation of biographical disruption. Soc. Sci. Med. 225, 120–127.

Faircloth, C.A., Boylstein, C., Rittman, R., Young, M.E., Gubrium, J., 2004. Sudden illness and biographical flow in narratives of stroke recovery. Sociol. Health Illn. 26(2), 242–261.

Liamputtong, P., Suwankhong, D., 2015. Breast cancer diagnosis: biographical disruption, emotional experiences and strategic management in Thai women with breast cancer. Sociol. Health Illn., 37(7), 1086–1101.

Locock, L., Ziebland, S., Dumelow, C., 2009. Biographical disruption, abruption, and repair in the context of motor neuron disease. Sociol. Health Illn. 31(7), 1043–1058.

Perry, B.L., Pescosolido, B.A., 2012. Social network dynamics and biographical disruption: the case of 'first-timers' with mental illness. Am. J. Sociol. 118(1), 134–175.

Sanderson, T., Calnan, M., Morris, M., Richards, P., Hewlett, S., 2011. Shifting normalities: interactions of changing conceptions of a normal life and the normalization of symptoms in rheumatoid arthritis. Sociol. Health Illn. 33(4), 618–633.

Saunders B., 2017. 'It seems like you're going around in circles': recurrent biographical disruption constructed through the past, present and anticipated future in the narratives of young adults with inflammatory bowel disease. Sociol. Health Illn. 39(5), 726–740. doi:10.1111/1467-9566.12561.

destination, the family decided to take her home. The disagreement created delays because no plans had been put in place to support a home discharge—as this option was not favoured by health and social services staff. In the following data extract (Case Study 3.2), we can see how these tensions are played out in the multidisciplinary team meeting, in which health and social services staff produce negative formulations of the family and their engagement with discharge planning processes.

CASE STUDY 3.2	Discharge Planning for Rosa Jackson

The ward manager shuffled the files about and then called out Rosa Jackson's name loudly and the conversations came to a halt.

Ward manager: After much umming and aahing the family now want her home, they had accepted nursing home about 2 weeks ago – err – sort of changed their minds want home, em, they want Rosa to return to the granddaughter's home, that is what we are working towards. OT (Occupational Thera-pist) is ordering a hoist, commode blah blah blah…
Consultant: This is the one who has several daughters?
Ward manager: No, one daughter, one son, couple of grandchildren.
Consultant: Yeah, but this is what I'm saying, there has been several (…)
Ward manager: Yeah, that's right
Occupational therapist: There's going to be a delay with the equipment, you know they're going to want home care, they'll need a bed I suppose, we haven't got a bed.
Consultant: Have they definitely decided to take her?
Occupational therapist: They are going to come up on Monday to spend a day looking after her.
Ward manager: (…) the family go away to America…
Doctor: What the granddaughter who is going to look after her?
Ward manager: Yeah!
Doctor: The granddaughter who is going to look after her is going to America!
Occupational therapist: Yeah
Doctor: For how long?
Occupational therapist: Two weeks (…) they've strung this out really, they knew the equipment was going to take a while to get
Consultant: If it's going to take a while, she should go into a nursing home until it's ready
Occupational therapist: Yeah, what about that for a…
Doctor: I told them last week that she is now ready to leave hospital and where she goes is not really relevant but she's now ready to leave hospital, she either goes home or to a nursing home, we need the bed
Social worker: I thought they had made up their minds, about a nursing home
Doctor: What we're saying is that they've procrastinated and now there is another delay of….
Consultant: Why I mean, did they delay for months?
Social worker: The granddaughter see, she's…
Consultant: I think we say she should go into a nursing home and then they will probably say, I don't know.
Occupational therapist: You know, I can, you know, book, order the equipment.
Consultant: Is there a place in the nursing home social worker?
Social worker: Well, if you look, yeah
Consultant: Funding?
Social worker: List. But I put her on the funding list quite a long time ago
Consultant: So that might have come through?
Social worker: Yeah, probably, I would imagine
Consultant: Well I think she should go into nursing home and then she will transfer to her own home which will take time because we will put in those requests
Occupational therapist: Yeah, I will order them, I'll order them
Consultant: Yes, fine she can go to her home in few months, but meantime she can go to a nursing home

With prmission from Allen, D., Griffiths, L., Lyne, P., Monaghan, L., Murphy D., 2000. Delivering Health and So-cial Care: Changing Roles, Responsibilities and Relationships. Final Report Submitted to the Welsh Office of Research and Development for Health and Social Care. ISBN: 1 903847 079. (meeting tape GM0915).

EXERCISE 3.6

Review Case Study 3.1 to consider how the 'people' element of Gareth Williams' care impacted on his recovery trajectory.
You can record your answer in the Care Trajectory Management Workbook (see Evolve website).

Take some time to reflect on this scenario before moving on to Exercise 3.6.

COMPLEXITY 6: HEALTHCARE IS CHARACTERISED BY MULTIPLE INSTITUTIONAL LOGICS

Healthcare, like many other organisations, is characterised by multiple institutional logics. An institutional logic provides a set of assumptions, beliefs and values that guide activity (Thornton and Ocasio, 1999). They are reflected in an organisation's material practices, work cultures and symbolic representations, and condition action by steering the attention of decision makers. It is not uncommon for multiple institutional logics to coexist in an organisation, and this can produce ambiguous or conflicting messages and formats that need to be managed in practice (Andersson and Liff, 2018; Goodrick and Reay, 2011). By focusing on the different logics that are present in a situation, we can understand some of the dynamics, dilemmas and experiences of professional practice. For example, professional logics emphasise practice focused on the individual needs of patients, whereas management logics focus on organisational standards and efficiency. Logics of recovery have a different emphasis from logics of comfort and palliation, and, as we have seen in the preceding section, the patient and their family have their own logic in utilising healthcare services which may not be in alignment with the prevailing logics of healthcare professionals. In certain contexts, institutional logics can be in tension, and in others they can coexist or even be mutually reinforcing (see Box 3.8 for some examples from healthcare). Nurses often find themselves at the intersection of different logics and have an important role in mediating these relationships (Allen, 2004; Chambliss, 1997; Kristiansen et al., 2016) (Exercise 3.7).

BOX 3.8 ■ Multiple Institutional Logics in Healthcare

Implementation of The Productive Ward

The Productive Ward: Releasing Time to Care is a quality improvement intervention developed by the National Health Service (NHS) in the United Kingdom. The intervention was informed by lean thinking, a set of management practices intended to sustain customer satisfaction but eliminate waste. The aim of The Productive Ward was to help NHS staff to improve productivity and reduce inefficiencies, with the aim of providing better quality, safer care and a better experience for patients and staff.

van den Broek et al. (2014) carried out a study to explore the implementation of The Productive Ward in a Dutch hospital. The authors illustrate how The Productive Ward is a hybrid intervention which combines a management logic (productivity) with a professional logic (releasing time to care). They explored the implementation of The Productive Ward in two wards that were piloting the intervention. They collected data through interviews with participants in the intervention (project leaders, project team members and workgroup members, including nurses, hospital director, communication advisor and external consultant), two focus groups undertaken with each pilot ward where data were generated through a guided discussion in a group (nurses, managers and internal advisors) and observations of project steering group meetings.

They discovered that while some participants referred to both management and professional logics simultaneously in describing The Productive Ward, the motives relating to a professional logic were more evident in the responses of nursing staff, while managers and directors were more likely to evoke a business logic. The authors suggest that this might reflect how the intervention was introduced to different groups across the organisation, with the professional logics being highlighted in communications to nursing staff and the business logic emphasised in communications with managers and directors.

The authors argued that while this 'double labelling' supported the introduction of the intervention, it eventually backfired when very limited additional time to care was released and nurses had little scope to exercise the autonomy to make changes promised by the programme. While at the beginning of the project nurses embraced the initiative with enthusiasm, this waned over the implementation process in the absence of concrete gains in terms of time released to care.

Continued

BOX 3.8 ■ Multiple Institutional Logics in Healthcare—cont'd

Different Logics Mean Different Actions

Logics have important implications for patient care and can point to different actions for the purposes of care and treatment. Consider the following example:

While working as an agency nurse on a medical ward in a large teaching hospital, I was assigned responsibility for patients in a six-bedded bay. I was informed that one of the patients was at the end of life and a 'do not attempt resuscitation' (DNAR) order was in place. On entering the bay after handover, the bedside curtains were drawn around the end-of-life patient, and family members were present. I introduced myself, and as there were no immediate nursing care requirements, I left the family, to check on the other patients. A few minutes later, one of the family members approached me and said they believed their loved one had passed away: 'he has gone'. They were not unduly distressed as the death was expected. I went to the bedside and was able to confirm that this was the case. I spent a few minutes comforting the family, drew the curtains fully around the bed to afford them some privacy while they spent time together and then left the ward area to inform the nurse in charge. The nurse in charge duly informed the junior doctor. As soon as this information was shared, the junior doctor went immediately to assess the patient and, unaware of the DNAR order, ushered the family away from the bed area, pulled the emergency bell and began resuscitation. This action had devastating effects on what was a peaceful and anticipated death, in which the family were able to be with their loved one to say their goodbyes and comfort each other. This incident happened in 1989 and yet I can remember it as if was yesterday.

---

van den Broek, J., Boselie, P., Paauwe, J., 2014. Multiple institutional logics in health care: 'Productive Ward: Releasing Time to Care'. Public Manag. Rev. 16, 1–20. doi:10.1080/14719037.2013.770059.

EXERCISE 3.7

After discharge from hospital, and despite his wife's efforts, Gareth was reluctant to follow a diabetic diet to manage his blood glucose levels. This was related to his depression. What logics are involved in the compromises that were reached in managing this scenario in the immediate period following discharge?

You can record your answer in the Care Trajectory Management Workbook (see Evolve website).

COMPLEXITY 7: HEALTHCARE REQUIRES BALANCING THE NEEDS OF THE INDIVIDUAL WITH THE NEEDS OF THE MANY

Although in healthcare the emphasis is on the requirements of individuals, patient care takes place within systems responsible for whole populations, whether in the hospital or the community. Meeting the needs of individuals must be balanced with the requirement to meet the needs of others within available resources. Compared to a factory or a hotel, care organisations have less control over their workflow and so experience constant churn and fluctuations in demand relating to the volume and intensity of patient care work and available capacity. This was evident on a global scale during the COVID-19 pandemic where shifts in the volume and patterns of demand necessitated radical reconfiguration of services and healthcare utilisation reduced by about a third, with greater decreases in people with less severe illness (Moynihan et al., 2021) (Box 3.9).

While COVID-19 is an extreme example, mechanisms of prioritisation are threaded throughout everyday healthcare practices, in the operation of waiting lists (Daniels and Sabin, 2002), the management of referral processes (Hughes and Griffiths, 1997), in formalised systems of triage (Mackway-Jones et al., 2014; Wilkinson, 2021) and in the everyday decisions taken by individual care providers about how best to deploy time and energy in the face of competing demands (Ball et al., 2014; Scott et al., 2019) (Box 3.10). Nurses, like other healthcare workers, frequently are responsible for a caseload of patients and must manage resources in meeting the needs of individuals under their care. While models of one-to-one care exist, these are the

---

BOX 3.9 ■ Impact of the COVID-19 Pandemic on Utilisation of Healthcare Services

Moynihan et al. (2021) undertook the first broad synthesis of global studies of COVID-19 pandemic-related changes in healthcare use across all categories of services. The review included 81 studies involving over 17.9 million services provided across 20 countries which reported estimates of changes in healthcare utilisation between pandemic and prepandemic. There was consistent evidence of reductions in the use of health services during the pandemic period up to May 2020. These findings were categorised into four main types of change: change in health visits, changes in healthcare admissions, changes in therapeutics and preventive care and changes in diagnostics.

The authors report that there was a consistent message across all the studies of the need for monitoring of the long-term impacts of missed care, public health campaigns to ensure people seek medical care when they need it and the requirement for better preparedness for reducing the extent of missed care in future waves of the pandemic. They argue that the evidence of excess population mortality, in addition to deaths from COVID-19, underlines the importance of these recommendations. At the same time, the review also identified that reductions in the use of health services were greater for less severe forms of illness, which, combined with some evidence about overprescribing, suggests that for some people missing care may not have caused harm. The authors conclude:

This unprecedented pandemic-induced natural experiment in reduced healthcare utilisation provides a genuine opportunity to learn more about what services populations and healthcare systems came to regard as lesser priorities, when redistribution of resources towards more essential services was needed to minimise mortality in a crisis. […] [G]reatly reduced ED attendances around the world for non-urgent complaints indicate an opportunity to inform and implement new strategies and models of care that maximise the appropriateness of visits in the future. […] Addressing genuine unmet need and winding back the harm and waste of unnecessary care are not conflicting interests, but rather two sides of a coherent strategy to efficiently improve human health.

(Moynihan et al., 2021, pp. 8–9).

With permission from Moynihan, R., Sanders, S., Michaleff, Z.A., Scott, A.M., Clark, J., To, E.J., et al., 2021. Impact of COVID-19 on utilisation of healthcare services: a systematic review. BMJ Open. 11, e045343. doi:10.1136/bmjopen-2020-045343.

EXERCISE 3.8

Return to Case Study 3.1 and review Gareth Williams' care from the point of admission home, how has his care been shaped by health services resource management, and prioritisation processes? You can record your answer in the Care Trajectory Management Workbook (see Evolve website).

exception rather than the rule. Consider the resource impacts on Gareth Williams' care by completing Exercise 3.8.

An Introduction to Complex Adaptive Systems

Considering the individual sources of healthcare complexity as we have done here is useful for learning purposes. In the real world of practice, however, these factors interact to generate a level of complexity which is far more than the sum of the individual parts. In recognition of this, there is a growing body of researchers and policy analysts who maintain that healthcare organisations should be understood as complex adaptive systems (Braithwaite, 2018; McDaniel and Driebe, 2001). The idea of a complex adaptive system draws on insights from complexity science, which asserts that some systems have qualities which cannot be understood by analysis of the individual parts. The most common definition of a complex adaptive system is a dynamic network of agents acting in parallel, constantly reacting to what the other agents are doing, which in turn influences individual behaviour and the overall network (Holland, 1992, cited by The Health Foundation, 2010).

BOX 3.10 ■ 'Care Left Undone' During Nursing Shifts

There is a growing body of international evidence which demonstrates an association between nurse staffing and patient outcomes. A systematic review of 102 studies concluded that increased registered nurse (RN) staffing levels are associated with lower rates of hospital mortality and adverse patient events (Kane et al., 2007). Despite the strength of evidence for a link between nurse staffing and clinical outcomes, relatively little is known about the mechanisms through which variations in nurse staffing impact on mortality, or other patient outcomes (Bolton et al., 2007).

Ball et al. (2014) carried out a study to explore whether 'missed care' could explain the relationship between nurse staffing and patient outcomes. The research involved a cross-sectional survey of a sample of surgical and medical wards in UK National Health Service general acute hospital Trusts (the bodies managing one or more hospitals) in England. The questionnaire included sections on work environment and job satisfaction, quality and safety, your recent shift, about you and where you work. Nurse staffing was calculated by asking nurses to report the staff giving direct patient care (specifically RN and other nursing care staff) and the number of patients on the ward on the last shift they worked. The nurses' work environment was assessed using the Practice Environment Scale (PES) of the Nursing Work Index, an internationally validated measure. The PES measures organisational factors—such as management support for nursing, doctor–nurse relationship and promotion of quality of care—which enhance or attenuate the nurse's ability to deliver high-quality care. Care left undone was assessed by asking nurses to indicate from a list of 13 items any care left unfinished because they did not have time to complete them in their most recent shift. These were:

- adequate patient surveillance
- adequate documentation of nursing care
- administering medication on time
- comfort/talk with patients
- develop or update nursing care plans/care pathways
- educating patients and/or family
- frequent changing of patient's position
- oral hygiene
- pain management
- planning care
- preparing patients and families for discharge
- skin care
- undertaking treatments/procedures

A total of 2917 responses were received from RNs in the medical and surgical wards.

The relationship between missed care and other variables (staffing level and practice environment) was explored through statistical modelling techniques. Most nurses working on general medical and surgical wards in this representative sample reported that some care was left undone on their last shift. Care that was frequently left undone included adequate patient surveillance, which has been hypothesised as a key mechanism explaining the association between low nurse staffing and increased mortality. The amount of care left undone was strongly related to nurses' overall perceptions of the quality and safety of care. The research findings revealed that nurses are more likely to report care being left undone (or 'missed') when they are working on shifts with high numbers of patients per RN. The number of activities left undone is also greater. Care is more likely to be left undone in wards where nurses perceive the practice environment to be worse.

Ball, J.E., Murrells, T., Rafferty, A.M., Morrow, E., Griffiths, P., 2014. 'Care left undone' during nursing shifts: associations with workload and perceived quality of care. BMJ Qual. Saf. 23, 116–125.
Bolton, L., Aydin, C., Donaldson, N., Brown, D.S., Sandhu, M., Fridman, M., et al., 2007. Mandated nurse staffing ratios in California: a comparison of staffing and nursing-sensitive outcomes pre- and post regulation. Policy Polit. Nurs. Pract. 8, 238–250.
Kane, R., Shamliyan, T., Mueller, C., Duval, S., Wilt, T.J., 2007. The association of registered nurse staffing levels and patient outcomes: systematic review and meta-analysis. Med. Care. 45, 1195–204.

In complex adaptive systems, control tends to be dispersed and decentralised and the overall behaviour of the system is the result of many decisions made constantly by individual agents (Waldrop, 1994, cited by The Health Foundation, 2010); order emerges rather than being predetermined. Employees who work in complex adaptive systems face high levels of uncertainty in their daily work (Braithwaite, 2018; McDaniel and Driebe, 2001). Nowhere is this more evident than in healthcare.

> *Healthcare is a complex adaptive system, meaning that the system's performance and behaviour changes over time and cannot be completely understood by simply knowing about the individual components. No other system is more complex: not banking, education, manufacturing, or the military. No other industry or sector has the equivalent range and breadth—such intricate funding models, the multiple moving parts, the complicated clients with diverse needs, and so many options and interventions for any one person's needs. Patient presentation is uncertain, and many clinical processes need to be individualised to each patient. Healthcare has numerous stakeholders, with different roles and interests, and uneven regulations that tightly control some matters and barely touch others. The various combinations of care, activities, events, interactions, and outcomes are, for all intents and purposes, infinite.*
>
> Braithwaite (2018, p. 1)

While the application of these ideas to healthcare is very recent, understanding healthcare organisations as complex adaptive systems has important implications for how we approach quality and safety, how we intervene to bring about improvements, how we understand the organisation and coordination of patient care and how we situate nursing's care trajectory management role.

Summary

This chapter has explored the qualities of healthcare work which contribute to the complexity of care trajectories: the highly specialised division of labour and the distributed nature of practice; healthcare's status as people work and the accumulative complexity and unpredictability of many illness and disease processes; the influence of multiple institutional logics and the challenges of balancing the needs of individuals with that of whole populations; and the impacts of the dynamic technological landscape on healthcare work. These sources of complexity are more than additive; they interact to create complex and turbulent care delivery environments, make care processes unpredictable and the organisation of care very difficult. The next chapter will explore different approaches to healthcare organisation and how these relate to care trajectory management.

SUMMARY OF KEY LEARNING

- Healthcare is a complex system of work, which can lead to unpredictable trajectories of care and create turbulent work environments.
- The seven complexities of healthcare work include its complex division of labour, the unpredictability of disease and illness processes, its status as people work, the existence of multiple institutional logics, its technological complexity, the distributed nature of practice and the requirement to balance the need of individuals with the needs of the many.
- The interactive effects of these sources of system complexity create high levels of organisational uncertainty.
- New research in which healthcare is conceptualised as a complex adaptive system has important implications for the understanding of quality and safety, approaches to service improvements and the organisation and coordination of care.

QUICK QUIZ

- What are the seven complexities of healthcare work?
- Why did Melia argue that simply measuring the tasks involved in patient care missed many of the activities and skills involved in hospital nursing?
- What does it mean to describe healthcare as a 'collective endeavour'?
- What is burden of treatment theory?
- What is meant by 'technology' in understanding healthcare work?
- Why can the term 'teamwork' be a misleading description of healthcare?
- What is the cumulative complexity model?
- What is biographical disruption?
- What is biographical flow?
- What is an institutional logic?
- What is a complex adaptive system?

References

Allen, D., 2000. Negotiating the role of expert carers on an adult hospital ward. Sociol. Health Illn. 22 (2), 149–171. doi:10.1111/1467-9566.00197.

Allen, D., 2004. Re-reading nursing and re-writing practice: towards an empirically based reformulation of the nursing mandate. Nurs. Inq. 11 (4), 271–283.

Allen, D., 2015. The Invisible Work of Nurses: Hospitals, Organisation and Healthcare. Routledge, London and New York.

Allen, D., 2016. The importance, challenges and prospects of taking work practices into account for healthcare quality improvement. J. Health Organ. Manag. 30 (4), 672–689. doi:10.1108/JHOM-04-2014-0062.

Allen, D., Griffiths, L., Lyne, P., Monaghan, L., Murphy D., 2000. Delivering Health and Social Care: Changing Roles, Responsibilities and Relationships. Final Report Submitted to the Welsh Office of Research and Development for Health and Social Care. ISBN: 1 903847 079.

Andersson, T., Liff, R., 2018. Co-optation as a response to competing institutional logics: professionals and managers in healthcare. J. Prof. Organ. 34 (4), 212–218.

Aveling, E., Parker, M., Dixon-Woods, M., 2016. What is the role of individual accountability in patient safety? A multi-site ethnographic study. Sociol. Health Illn. 38 (2), 216–232.

Ball, J.E., Murrells, T., Rafferty, A.M., Morrow, E., Griffiths, P., 2014. 'Care left undone' during nursing shifts: associations with workload and perceived quality of care. BMJ Qual. Saf. 23, 116–125.

Benner, P., 1984. From Novice to Expert: Excellence and Power in Clinical Nursing Practice. Addison-Wesley Publishing Company, Menlo Park, CA.

Benner, P., Tanner, C., 1987. Clinical judgment: how expert nurses use intuition. Am. J. Nurs. 1, 23–31.

Berg, M., 1997. Rationalising Medical Work: Decision Support Technologies and Medical Practice. MIT, Cambridge, MA.

Bourdieu, P., 1980. The Logic of Practice. Stanford University Press, Stanford.

Braithwaite, J., 2018. Changing how we think about healthcare improvement. Br. Med. J. 361, 1–5. doi:10.1136/bmj.k2014.

Bury, M., 1982. Chronic illness as biographical disruption. Sociol. Health Illn. 4 (2), 167–182.

Chambliss, D., 1997. Beyond Caring: Hospitals, Nurses, and the Social Organization of Ethics. University of Chicago Press, Chicago, IL.

Corbin, J., Strauss, A., 1988. Unending Work and Care: Managing Chronic Illness at Home. Jossey-Bass Inc., San Fransisco, CA.

Daniels, N., Sabin, J.E., 2002. Setting Limits Fairly. Oxford University Press, Oxford.

Dent, M., 1990. Organisation and change in renal work: a study of the impact of a computer system within two hospitals. Sociol. Health Illn. 12 (4), 413–431.

Dingwall, R., Allen, D., 2001. The implications of healthcare reforms for the profession of nursing. Nurs. Inq. 8 (2), 64–74.

Ellingsen, G., Monteiro, E., 2003. Mechanisms for producing a working knowledge: enacting, orchestrating and organizing. Inform. Organ. 13, 203–229.

Goodrick, E., Reay, T., 2011. Constellations of institutional logics: changes in the professional work of pharmacists. Work Occup. 38 (3), 372–416.

Hannigan, B., Allen, D., 2013. Complex caring trajectories in community mental health: contingencies, divisions of labor and care coordination. Commun. Ment. Health J. 49 (4), 380–388. doi:10.1007/s10597-011-9467-9.

Hansten, R., Washburn, M., 2000. Intuition in professional practice: executive and staff perceptions. J. Nurs. Adm. 30 (4), 185–189.

Hardey, M., Payne, S., Coleman, P., 2000. 'Scraps' hidden nursing information and its influence on the delivery of care. J. Adv. Nurs. 32 (1), 208–214.

Heath, C., 1982. Preserving the consultation: medical record charts and professional conduct. Sociol. Health Illn. 4 (1), 56–74.

Heath, C., Luff, P., Svensson, M.S., 2003. Technology and medical practice. Sociol. Health Illn. 25 (3), 75–96.

Holland, J.H., 1992. Adaptation in Natural and Artificial Systems: An Introductory Analysis With Applications to Biology, Control, and Artificial Intelligence. MIT Press, Cambridge, MA.

Hughes, D., Griffiths, L., 1997. 'Ruling in' and 'ruling out': two approaches to the micro-rationing of healthcare. Soc. Sci. Med. 44 (5), 589–599.

Hutchins, E., 1995. Cognition in the Wild. MIT Press, Cambridge, MA.

Kassahun, W.T., 2018. The effects of pre-existing dementia on surgical outcomes in emergent and nonemergent general surgical procedures: assessing differences in surgical risk with dementia. BMC Geriatr. 18 (1), 153. doi:10.1186/s12877-018-0844-x.

Kristiansen, M., Obstfelder, A., Lotherington, A.T., 2016. Contradicting logics in everyday practice. J. Health Organ. Manag. 30 (1), 57–72.

Lin, C.S., Chang, C.C., Lee, Y.W., Liu, C.C., Yeh, C.C., Chang, Y.C., et al., 2019. Adverse outcomes after major surgeries in patients with diabetes: a multicenter matched study. J. Clin. Med. 8 (1), 100. doi:10.3390/jcm8010100.

Mackway-Jones, K., Marsden, J., Windle, J., 2014. Emergency Triage: Manchester Triage Group, third ed. BMJ Books, Cowley Oxford.

May, C.R., Eton, D.T., Boehmer, K., Gallacher, K., Hunt, K., MacDonald, S., et al., 2014. Rethinking the patient: using Burden of Treatment Theory to understand the changing dynamics of illness. BMC Health Serv. Res. 14 (281). doi:10.1186/1472-6963-14-281.

McDaniel, R.R., Driebe, D.J., 2001. Complexity Science and Health Care Management (Advances in Health Care Management, Vol. 2). Emerald Group Publishing Limited, Bingley, pp. 11–36.

Melia, K.M., 1979. A sociological approach to the analysis of nursing work. J. Adv. Nurs. 4, 57–67.

Mental Health Foundation, 2022. Long-term physical conditions and mental health. https://www.mental-health.org.uk/explore-mental-health/a-z-topics/long-term-physical-conditions-and-mental-health (Accessed 19 July 2022).

Moynihan, R., Sanders, S., Michaleff, Z.A., Scott, A.M., Clark, J., To, E.J., et al., 2021. Impact of COVID-19 on utilisation of healthcare services: a systematic review. BMJ Open 11, e045343. doi:10.1136/bmjopen-2020-045343.

Pilnick, A., 2022. Reconsidering Patient Centred Care: Between Autonomy and Abandonment. Emerald Publishing Limited, Bingley, UK.

Pilnick, A., Dingwall, R., 2011. On the remarkable persistence of asymmetry in doctor/patient interaction: a critical review. Soc. Sci. Med. 72 (8), 1374–1382. doi:10.1016/j.socscimed.2011.02.033.

Prout, A., 1996. Actor-network theory, technology and medical sociology: an illustrative analysis of the metered dose inhaler. Sociol. Health Illn. 18 (2), 198–219.

Sandelowski, M., 2000. Devices & Desires: Gender, Technology and American Nursing. The University of North Carolina Press, Chapel Hill, NC.

Schmidt, K., Simone, C., 1996. Coordination mechanisms: towards a conceptual foundation of CSCW systems design. Comput. Support Coop. Work 5, 155–200.

Scott, A.P., Harvey, C., Felzmann, H., Suhonen, R., 2019. Resource allocation and rationing in nursing care: a discussion paper. Nurs. Ethics 26 (5), 1528–1539.

Shippee, N.D., Shah, N.D., May, C.R., Mair, F.S., Montori, V.M., 2012. Cumulative complexity: a functional, patient-centred model of patient complexity can improve research and practice. J. Clin. Epidemiol. 65, 1041–1051.

The Health Foundation, 2010. Evidence Scan: Complex Adaptive Systems. The Health Foundation, London.

The Health Foundation and the King's Fund, 2015. Making Change Possible: A Transformation Fund for the NHS. The Health Foundation, London.

Thornton, P.H., Ocasio, W., 1999. Institutional logics and the historical contingency of power in organizations: executive succession in the higher education publishing Industry, 1958–1990. Am. J. Sociol. 105 (3), 801–843.

Timmermans, S., Berg, M., 2003. The practice of medical technology. Sociol. Health Illn. 25 (3), 97–114.

Waldrop, M.M., 1994. Complexity: The Emerging Science at the Edge of Order and Chaos. Penguin, Harmondsworth, London.

Wilkinson, D.J.C., 2021. Frailty triage: is rationing intensive medical treatment on the grounds of frailty ethical? Am. J. Bioeth. 21 (11), 48–63. doi:10.1080/15265161.2020.1851809.

WHO, 2018. Assistive Technology. https://www.who.int/news-room/fact-sheets/detail/assistive-technology (Accessed 30 November 2022).

Winance, M., 2006. Trying out the wheelchair: the mutual shaping of people and devices through adjustment. Sci. Technol. Hum. Values 31 (1), 52–72.

Suggested Reading

Family Carers

Allen, D., 2000. Negotiating the role of expert carers on an adult hospital ward. Sociol. Health Illn. 22 (2), 149–171. doi:10.1111/1467-9566.00197.

Exley, C., Allen, D., 2007. A critical examination of home care: end of life care as an illustrative case. Soc. Sci. Med. 65 (11), 2317–2327.

Lowes, L., Lyne, P., 2001. Chronic sorrow in parents of children with newly diagnosed diabetes: a review of the literature and discussion of the implications for nursing practice. J. Adv. Nurs. 32 (1), 41–48. doi:10.1046/j.1365-2648.2000.01418.x.

Some examples of studies which illustrate how illness impacts carers and the implications this has for the organisation of work.

Biographical Disruption

Bell, S.L., Tyrrell, J., Phoenix, C., 2016. Ménière's disease and biographical disruption: where family transitions collide. Soc. Sci. Med. 166, 177–185. doi:10.1016/j.socscimed.2016.08.025.

Harden, J., 2005. Parenting a young person with mental health problems: temporal disruption and reconstruction. Sociol. Health Illn. 27 (3), 351–371.

Some further examples of studies of biographical disruption.

Balancing the Needs of Individuals With the Needs of Many

Albrecht, G., 2001. Rationing healthcare to disabled people. Sociol. Health Illn. 23 (5), 654–677.

Allan, H.T., 2000. A 'good enough' nurse: supporting patients in a fertility clinic. Nurs. Inq. 8, 51–60.

Allen, D., Griffiths, L., Lyne, P., 2004. Accommodating health and social care needs: routine resource allocation in stroke rehabilitation. Sociol. Health Illn. 26 (4), 411–432. doi:10.1111/j.0141-9889.2004.00397.x.

Hillman, A., 2014. Why must I wait? The performance of legitimacy in a hospital emergency department. Sociol. Health Illn. 36 (4), 485–499.

Purkis, M.E., 1996. Nursing in quality space: technologies governing experiences of care. Nurs. Inq. 3 (2), 101–111.

A selection of observational studies which have documented everyday process of managing demands for care within available resources.

Institutional Logics

ten Dam, E.M., Waardenburg, M., 2020. Logic fluidity: how frontline professionals use institutional logics in their day-to-day work. J. Prof. Organ. 7 (2), 188–204. doi:10.1093/jpo/joaa012.

A study of institutional logics.

Complex Adaptive Systems Thinking

Braithwaite, J., Churruca, K., Ellis, L.A., Long, J., Clay-Williams, R., Damen, N., et al., 2017. Complexity Science in Healthcare – Aspirations, Approaches, Applications and Accomplishments: A White Paper. Australian Institute of Health Innovation. Macquarie University, Sydney, Australia. https://www.mq.edu.au/__data/assets/pdf_file/0012/683895/Braithwaite-2017-Complexity-Science-in-Healthcare-A-White-Paper-1.pdf.

An accessible and engaging overview of developments in complexity science and their implications for healthcare.

Approaches to Organising Healthcare

LEARNING OUTCOMES

At the end of this chapter, you will be able to:
- Describe rational–linear approaches to organisation
- Describe emergent approaches to organisation
- Describe the relationship between rational–linear and emergent approaches in healthcare
- Describe how rational–linear and emergent approaches are combined in care trajectory management

Introduction

This chapter builds on Chapter 3 to explore the implications of the complexities of healthcare work for organising patient care. It will consider two approaches to managing complex processes: the rational–linear model of organisation and the emergent model of organisation. Care trajectory management involves both rational–linear and emergent approaches, and the ability to adopt the most appropriate model to the requirements of the situation.

Rational–Linear Organisation

In recent history the dominant response to the organisational challenges of healthcare has been the use of rational–linear models of organising underpinned by ideas from the fields of engineering and management science. Rational–linear approaches treat organisations as if they were machines; they assume that if the individual components of the organisation are understood, then it is possible to understand the whole and, if each part of the organisation can be made to work better, then the whole organisation will work better too. Rational–linear approaches privilege planning, standardisation, guidelines, and structural solutions to the challenges of organisation. While the origins of this approach can be traced to the classical management theory of the late 19th century (Fayol, 1949), probably one of its most well-known manifestations is in the scientific management principles of the 1920s applied by Frederick Taylor to the production processes at The Ford Motor Company and which led to the creation of assembly lines that made standardisation and mass production possible (Taylor, 1911). The approach has undergone several incarnations in the intervening period—such as Total Quality Management of the 1980s (Martínez-Lorente et al., 1998), the business process reengineering of the 1990s (Hammer and Champy, 1993) and lean management of the 2000s (Womack and Jones, 1996)—but the core ideas remain deeply embedded in organisational theory and management science.

Rational–linear approaches have become increasingly widespread in healthcare systems as acceptable strategies for the management of complex organisational processes. This includes large-scale service reengineering projects (McNulty and Ferlie, 2002), local implementation of lean management approaches (Waring and Bishop, 2010) and a plethora of interventions designed to manage clinical processes and coordinate activity (Gabbay and le May, 2004, 2011; Moreira, 2005; Pinder et al., 2005; Timmermans and Berg, 1997). The metaphor of the patient pathway described in Chapter 2 is an example of this way of thinking. Other examples with which you will be familiar include integrated care pathways (ICPs), clinical guidelines, protocols and decision-making algorithms (Allen, 2009). Work through Exercise 4.1 to stimulate your thinking.

EXERCISE 4.1

Write down a list of all the formal management processes you have experienced in healthcare practice. These can relate to the management of efficiency, patient flows or interventions to address quality and safety.

You can record your answer in the Care Trajectory Management Workbook (see Evolve website).

While healthcare and other organisations *behave* as if their internal processes can be controlled by rational–linear methods, to some extent this is a myth. Formal structures and rational processes are adopted as much for the purposes of legitimation as they are to address the intrinsic demands of the work. As Meyer and Rowan (1997) have shown, organisations seek societal support by incorporating structures and procedures that match widely accepted cultural models. They argue that, consequently, much of what happens in organisations stems not from the work requirements, but from symbols, beliefs and rituals.

> *By designing a formal structure that adheres to the prescription myths in the institutional environment, an organization demonstrates that it is acting on collectively valued purposes in a proper and adequate manner.*
>
> Meyer and Rowan (1977, p. 349)

Modern societies are dominated by norms of rationality which play a causal role in providing the templates for the design of organisations. In the face of growing concerns about quality and safety, the guidelines, checklists and protocols which have proliferated in healthcare over the past three decades can be understood as an attempt to signal to the outside world that the organisation takes its internal procedures seriously and is making a good faith effort to improve service processes. Indeed, as described in Chapter 1 in the example of risk assessments tools in older people (see Box 1.2), many of the formal management technologies that characterise healthcare systems are driven by the need to satisfy quality assurance processes imposed by external regulatory agencies (Allen, 2017). There is much to debate about the impact of these systems on the burgeoning volume of paperwork that healthcare professionals routinely complain about, and questions that could be asked about whether care is paper safe or really safe (Smith, 2018). For current purposes, however, the point to emphasise is that the dominance of rational–linear approaches in healthcare systems is the product not only of coordinative demands imposed by the complexity of patient care and treatment but also of cultural norms that legitimate the adoption of specific models or approaches for addressing these challenges. For the reasons outlined in the previous chapter, alternative forms of organising are also necessary to hold together patient care, but much of this activity goes on under the radar of formal organisational processes. See Box 4.1 for some critical insights.

BOX 4.1 ■ Insights From Critical Studies of Standardisation in Healthcare

Sociologists have offered insights which challenge the logic of standardisation in healthcare. Wiener (2000) examined efforts in the United States to increase hospital care quality through enhanced standardisation of work. Drawing on extensive observational work in two hospitals, she concludes that many aspects of care resist standardisation, and as such, standardisation in health will remain an elusive quest.

In the context of the English National Health Service, McDonald et al. (2006) explored the views of clinicians and managers on standardisation. They concluded these groups had not only vastly different identities, histories and characteristics but also entirely different worldviews. Doctors believed quality and safety were an art, and managers thought it was a science. While doctors opposed standardisation, advocated the legitimacy of clinical judgement and tolerated uncertainty and risk, managers sought standardisation and adherence to guidelines and believed that structured, linear, rational solutions could be successfully applied to complex socio-professional environments.

I studied the integrated care pathway community, through attending the annual conference over several years (Allen, 2010a, 2010b). One delegate, a senior nurse, shared her experiences of leading pathway development in the organisation. She confided that her enthusiasm for the methodology had been eroded by the realisation that her performance was to be measured by the number of pathways developed and implemented over a year, rather than the impact of care pathways on patient outcomes. Others shared atrocity tales of complex integrated pathways, months in development, being ceremonially burnt in waste paper bins by clinical staff who did not consider them to be fit for purpose.

Allen, D., 2010a. Care pathways: an ethnographic description of the field. Int. J. Care Pathw. 14(1), 4–9.
Allen, D., 2010b. Care pathways: some social scientific observations on the field. Int. J. Care Pathw. 14(2), 47–51.
McDonald, R., Waring, J., Harrison, S., 2006. Rules, safety and the narrativization of identity: a hospital operating theatre case study. Sociol. Health Illn. 28(2), 178–202.
Wiener, C., 2000. The Elusive Quest: Accountability in Hospitals. Aldine de Gruyter, Hawthorne, New York.

Emergent Organisation

In *Social Organization of Medical Work*, Strauss et al. (1985) drew attention to the emergent and uncertain qualities of patient care, comparing healthcare processes to the challenges faced by Mark Twain's celebrated Mississippi River pilot:

> *[T]he river was tricky, changed its course slightly from day-to-day, so even an experienced, but inattentive pilot could run into grave difficulties; worse yet, sometimes the river drastically shifted in its bed for some miles into a new course. [...] Some of the various contingencies may be anticipated, but only a portion of them may be relatively controllable, [...] stemming as they do, not only from the illnesses themselves but from organizational sources.*
>
> Strauss et al. (1985, pp. 19–20)

As well as stimulating the development of the illness trajectory concept (see Chapter 2: From Care Pathways to Care Trajectories), Strauss et al.'s observations on the nonlinear qualities of healthcare work laid the foundations for the development of the *negotiated order perspective* in which organisation is conceptualised as arising from flow and ordering processes. The negotiated order perspective was one of the first theories of emergent organisation. In contrast to rational–linear models, in which order is considered to be generated from the top down through structures, plans and procedures, in the 'emergent organising' approach, order is understood as developing from the bottom up in the interactions between participants as they make sense of and manage situations, conundrums and unexpected occurrences in their work (Allen, 2019).

EXERCISE 4.2

Review your answers to Exercise 4.1; now think about the circumstances in which these formal management processes break down in practice. What actions are necessary to overcome these challenges and what are the impacts on care processes?

Before reading further, work through this exercise. You can record your answer in the Care Trajectory Management Workbook (see Evolve website).

Emergent modes of organising are recognised as a legitimate and necessary response to the demands of managing complex and unpredictable work environments and are evident in a range of contexts in contemporary society, such as offshore software development (Boden et al., 2008), global engineering (Pernille and Christensen, 2011) and marketing (Kellogg et al., 2006). Rather than envisaging organisations as machines, emergent organisation understands organisations as dynamic ecologies, which shape shift as a result of the interactions between participants and the work environment. In contrast to rational–linear approaches, emergent organisation depends not on the application of standard processes and procedures, but on nuanced and contextualised professional judgements and negotiations between participants in response to contingencies (Exercise 4.2). In the context of the shift towards understanding healthcare as a complex adaptive system, there is a growing recognition that emergent models are an important mode of organising to meet the needs of healthcare environments in the 21st century.

The world moves quickly; baselines shift; technologies crash; actions are (variously) constrained; and certainty is elusive. The gap between the evidence-based ideal and the political and material realities of the here-and-now may be wide. Decisions must be made on the basis of incomplete or contested data. People use their creativity and generate adaptive solutions that make sense locally. The articulations, workarounds and muddling-through that keep the show on the road are not footnotes in the story, but its central plot.

Greenhalgh and Papoutsi (2018, p. 2)

The Relationship Between the Rational–Linear and Emergent Models of Organisation in Practice

Rational–linear and emergent approaches produce very different depictions of organisational processes. These can be illustrated by borrowing some images from ornithology. Rational–linear organisation has parallels with the elegant V-shaped flight formation of geese and other migratory birds, which improves their energy efficiency (Fig. 4.1).

Emergent organisation is more akin to the hypnotic shape-shifting murmuration of starlings as they twist and swoop across the sky (Fig. 4.2). It is thought that by offering safety in numbers, a murmuration affords protection from predators, and it is their extremely fast reaction times that enable starlings to make split-second changes to their flight direction that prevents them from crashing into each other (Country File, N.D.).

While we do not see geese and starlings flying together, in most organisations, rational–linear and emergent forms of organisation coexist. The organisation of some activities is exclusively linear or emergent; in certain circumstances, workers switch between operating modes, and sometimes organisation can take a hybrid form, blending the rational–linear and emergent in a variety of forms.

In the context of healthcare, this relationship can be fruitfully explored through the example of ICPs. An extension of the patient pathway maps explored in Chapter 2, ICPs are multidisciplinary care management tools which map out chronologically all activities in a healthcare process.

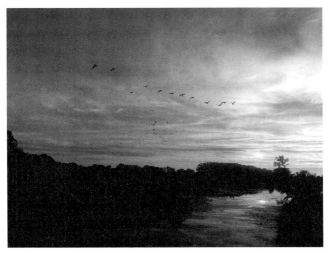

Fig. 4.1   Geese flying over Warner Park Lagoon. (From Wikimedia Commons Licence CC BY-SA 3.0.)

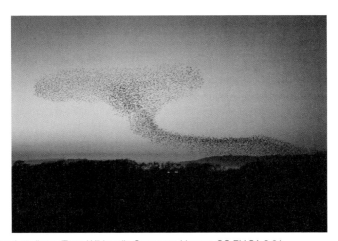

Fig. 4.2   Studland starlings. (From Wikimedia Commons Licence CC BY-SA 3.0.)

They are simultaneously a workflow system and a record of care. While originally developed as a tool for managing nursing care in North America (Pinder et al., 2005), enthusiasm for their use has spread across the world and they have been a feature of health systems for about 30 years. Like The Productive Ward (see Chapter 3, Box 3.8), ICPs are hybrid technologies which combine clinical and management logics in a single intervention. They have been promoted as a mechanism for creating partnerships between clinicians and managers, which helps to explain their growing popularity as quality improvement interventions to address the challenges of care coordination (Allen, 2010). ICPs specify the activities to be accomplished and require documentation to indicate compliance or noncompliance with planned interventions. ICP methodology acknowledges that not all patient care can be standardised in alignment with the prescriptions of the pathway, but any such 'deviation' is termed a 'variance', which must be recorded and explained in the documentation.

As the popularity of ICPs for improving care processes has grown, they have increasingly been selected as the intervention of choice to address coordination and standardisation processes in a wide range of contexts. I led a team which carried out a systematic review of the research evidence to explore the circumstances in which ICPs improved care coordination (Allen et al., 2009). The review focused on high-quality trials that evaluated the effectiveness of ICPs in both adult and child healthcare settings (1980–2008). The findings revealed that ICPs can be of value in improving care in clinical conditions and processes which follow a predictable course, particularly where interventions are time critical. However, in circumstances in which patient trajectories are less predictable and care must be tailored to the individual, then ICPs have limited value. While it is tempting to reach for rational–linear approaches to address service delivery challenges because these are the widely accepted models for managing an activity, and they bring with them the promise of order and control, this may not be an appropriate solution for the underlying organisational challenge.

As part of this research programme, we studied the development of an ICP for the rehabilitation of patients who had suffered a hip fracture (Allen, 2009, 2016). Pathway development was led by a quality improvement manager in collaboration with the clinical team as part of a wider effort to 'pathway' the whole patient trajectory from admission to discharge. While preoperative and postoperative care had been successfully mapped, and had been of value in aligning care processes, rehabilitation was challenging because of the high levels of variability in patient need. The rehabilitation pathway was eventually developed and implemented but failed to be embedded in practice because of its poor fit with the variability of healthcare processes. For staff at the point of service delivery, the pathway was primarily an elaborate document of care processes, rather than an aid to coordination, the work of which continued in the largely responsive way in which it had always been done. Interestingly, the hospital later appointed senior nurses to coordinate the hip fracture care trajectory, in what we might think of as a specialist care trajectory management role, in recognition, perhaps, of the limitations of rational models of organisation in this patient population which call for a more individualised approach founded on expert professional judgement. So, in selecting approaches to organising healthcare, it important to find the most appropriate model to the task at hand. Please see Box 4.2 for more examples. As Timmermans and Berg (2003) have argued:

[T]he issue is not for or against evidence-based medicine, guidelines or electronic patient records, but what shape they should take and how they should be put to work. A focus on the multiple

---

BOX 4.2 ■ Beyond Standardisation

Discretionary Practice in Face-to-Face Triage Nursing

The Manchester Triage System is a tool designed to manage clinical risk and prioritise care in conditions of limited capacity. It enables patients to be prioritised, based on signs and symptoms, without making any assumptions about the underlying diagnosis. It was developed by the Manchester Triage Group in 1997, which included physicians and nurses, and the aim was to organise the UK urgent care system and establish a consensus for a triage pattern (Mackway-Jones et al., 2014).

The Manchester Triage System comprises 55 flowcharts and uses a methodology that defines clinical priority by determining the maximum allowed waiting time for different levels of urgency: emergency (red) needs immediate medical evaluation, very urgent (orange) within 10 minutes, urgent (yellow) within 60 minutes, standard (green) within 120 minutes and nonurgent (blue) up to 240 minutes. It has since become one of the most used triage systems in Europe. The underlying logic is that more serious cases must have less waiting time for medical care and, therefore, shorter time to starting treatment.

Johannessen (2017) studied nurses' use of the Manchester Triage System in a Norwegian emergency primary care clinic (EPCC), using ethnographic research methods. A total of 349 face-to-face nursing assessments were observed in the EPCC, with further observations carried out in two other emergency services for comparative purposes. The data also included interviews with nurses, physicians and managers, and observations of mandatory training courses in nurse triage.

Johannessen describes how nurses assessed patients at odds with the Manchester Triage System by collecting supplementary information, performing differential and holistic reasoning, relying on emotion or intuition and allowing patients, relatives or colleagues to influence their decision making. In cases where nurses' own assessments indicated that the system-prescribed wait time was unreasonable, then nurses would workaround the system by qualifying discriminators, strategically choosing flowcharts or orally adjusting urgency levels.

Johannessen is at pains to emphasise that nurses did not simply disregard the Manchester Triage System guidelines. Rather, the Manchester Triage System served as a support system and checklist, holding nurses accountable to a minimum of symptoms and signs to be considered in their assessments and documentation. Nurses' assessments therefore synthesised their own professional judgement with system-prescribed considerations; rather than simply disregarding guidelines, they used them reflexively by drawing on some parts rather than others, supplementing or circumventing them when it was considered necessary to ensure fair and correct priority setting' (Johannessen, 2017, p. 1190).

Blended Implementation of a Surgical Care Pathway

Martin et al. (2017) examined the adoption and adaptation of a clinical pathway in emergency laparotomy. Implementation processes were studied using ethnographic methods (interviews, observation of site level meetings and forums and documentary analysis) as part of EPOCH, a large, randomised trial which included teams of surgeons and physicians in six sites in the UK. The researchers found near-universal receptivity to the concept of a pathway as a means of improving perioperative processes and outcomes, but also identified concerns about the impact on appropriate professional judgement. Rather than these concerns leading to resistance to the pathway, however, it resulted in a 'nuancing of the pathways-as-realised in each site'. On the one hand, the standardisation afforded by the pathway was seen as value in a 'forgotten group' of patients. On the other hand, there was concern about the limitations of standardisation in what was a heterogeneous population. Accordingly, those responsible for realising the pathway evolved from a logic of ensuring compliance with each node of the pathway towards a focus on those aspects that had an indirect impact on quality of care, by informing professional judgement rather than sidelining it. Martin et al.'s findings underline the importance of implementation processes in enabling a pathway to work in the complex world of healthcare practice. The authors conclude:

> Our findings suggest that, utilised in a reflexive, nuanced manner, pathways may have potential in championing and improving quality even outside the relatively linear, predictable patient groups and routines for which they were originally devised. This was underwritten by the approach taken by the core EPOCH team, which presented an evidence and consensus-based pathway, provided training in quality-improvement tools to help to achieve it, but left to the discretion of local teams the question of what components to prioritise, and how to realise them [...] What emerged were pathways-in-practice that, while still offering good-practice prescriptions, deferred to and valorised situated professional decision-making in the face of real-world ethical dilemmas – but also sought to improve the quality of that professional decision-making by encouraging the generation and use of supplementary information that could give rise to better judgements and better interactions among professional groups.
>
> (Martin et al., 2017, p. 1326)

Johannessen, L.E.F., 2017. Beyond guidelines: discretionary practice in face-to-face triage nursing. Sociol. Health Illn. 39(7), 1180–1194.

Mackway-Jones, K., Marsden, J., Windle, J., 2014. Emergency Triage/Manchester Triage Group, third edition. BMJ Books, Cowley Oxford.

Martin, G.P., Kocman, D., Stephens, T., Peden, C.J., Pearse, R.M., 2017. Pathways to professionalism? Quality improvement, care pathways, and the interplay of standardisation and clinical autonomy. Sociol. Health Illn. 39(8), 1314–1329.

goals and interests at stake and on the way standards have to be made to work is of vital importance here. A deep knowledge of the characteristics of health care work is crucial to be able to find the synergy between the standard's coordinating activity and the staff members' embodied expertise.

Timmermans and Berg (2003, p. 202)

Rational–Linear and Emergent Organisation in Care Trajectory Management

As the examples in Box 4.2 illustrate, in most complex systems, rational and emergent approaches to organisation coexist and expert care trajectory management requires the ability to combine and move between different modes of organising as required. This involves considered engagement with formal rational systems and processes as resources that support practice, rather than blind adherence or blatant noncompliance. The processes through which rational–linear and emergent forms of organisation are managed in practice can be understood as a form of sensemaking (Weick, 1995) and will be considered in subsequent chapters. Consolidate your learning in this chapter by completing Exercise 4.3.

EXERCISE 4.3

You have been approached to contribute to the development of an end-to-end pathway for stroke management. Return to Case Study 3.1 (Chapter 3) and think about the different stages of Gareth Williams' trajectory of care. Are there aspects of care and treatment that might usefully be managed by a pathway? Are there aspects of care and treatment where a pathway has less value? Explain the reasons for your answers.

You can record your answer in the Care Trajectory Management Workbook (see Evolve website).

Summary

This chapter has considered different approaches to organising healthcare and why emergent models of organisation underpinned by professional judgement are a necessary complement to rational–linear approaches informed by management science. These different modes of organising are combined in care trajectory management and will be explored further in forthcoming chapters.

SUMMARY OF KEY LEARNING

- Contemporary healthcare systems are dominated by rational–linear approaches to organisation, which render invisible the more responsive and emergent modes of organising that are necessary to respond to the unpredictable qualities of healthcare work.
- Emergent approaches to organisation are necessary in complex adaptive systems, where work processes are subject to high levels of uncertainty.
- Care trajectory management entails both rational–linear and emergent approaches to organisation and requires the ability to combine, nuance and move between different modes in response to the needs of the situation.

QUICK QUIZ

- What are the origins of rational–linear approaches to organisation?
- What are the origins of emergent approaches to organisation?
- What is the primary difference between rational–linear and emergent approaches to organisation?
- Why are rational–linear approaches an attractive solution to organisational challenges?
- What image from ornithology best depicts rational–linear approaches to organisation?
- What image from ornithology best depicts emergent approaches to organisation?
- Why does healthcare require both rational–linear and emergent approaches to organisation?
- Why do Greenhalgh and Papoutsi argue that the workarounds and muddling-through that keep the show on the road are not footnotes in the story, but its central plot?

References

Allen, D., 2009. From boundary concept to boundary object: the practice and politics of care pathway development. Soc. Sci. Med. 69 (3), 354–361.

Allen, D., 2010. Care pathways: an ethnographic description of the field. Int. J. Care Pathw. 14 (1), 4–9.

Allen, D., 2016. The importance, challenges and prospects of taking work practices into account for healthcare quality improvement. J. Health Organ. Manag. 30 (4), 672–689.

Allen, D., 2017. From polyformacy to formacology. BMJ Qual. Saf. 26 (9), 695–697.

Allen, D., 2019. Institutionalising emergent organisation in health and social care. J. Health Organ. Manag. 33 (7/8), 764–775.

Allen, D., Gillen, E., Rixson, L., 2009. A systematic review of the effectiveness of integrated care pathways: what works, for whom, in which circumstances?. Int. J. Evid. Based Healthc. 7, 61–74.

Boden, A., Nett, B., Wulf, V., 2008. Articulation work in small-scale offshore software development projects. Paper presented at the CHASE'08. Leipzig, Germany.

Country File, N.D. Starling murmuration guide: why and when they happen and best places to see one in the UK. https://www.countryfile.com/wildlife/birds/what-is-a-murmuration-and-where-are-the-best-places-in-britain-to-see-one/ (Accessed 30 November 2022).

Fayol, H., 1949. General and Industrial Management. Pitman, London.

Gabbay, J., le May, A., 2004. Evidence based guidelines or collectively constructed 'mindlines'? Ethnographic study of knowledge management in primary care. Br. Med. J. 329 (7473), 1249–1252.

Gabbay, J., le May, A., 2011. Practice-Based Evidence for Health Care: Clinical Mindlines. Routledge, Abingdon.

Greenhalgh, T., Papoutsi, C., 2018. Studying complexity in health services research: desperately seeking an overdue paradigm shift. BMC Med. 16 (95). doi:10.1186/s12916-018-1089-4.

Hammer, M., Champy, J., 1993. Re-Engineering the Corporation: A Manifesto for Business Revolution. Nicholas Brearley Publishing, London.

Kellogg, K., Orlikowski, W., Yates, J., 2006. Life in the trading zone: structuring coordination across boundaries in post bureaucratic organizations. Organ. Sci. 17, 22–44.

Martínez-Lorente, A.R., Dewhurst, F., Dale, B.G., 1998. Total quality management: origins and evolution of the term. The TQM Magazine 10 (5), 378–386. doi:10.1108/09544789810231261.

McNulty, T., Ferlie, E., 2002. Reengineering Healthcare: The Complexities of Organizational Transformation. Oxford University Press, Oxford.

Meyer, J.W., Rowan, B., 1977. Institutionalized organizations: formal structure as myth and ceremony. Am. J. Sociol. 83 (2), 340–363.

Moreira, T., 2005. Diversity in clinical guidelines: the role of repertoires of evaluation. Soc. Sci. Med. 60 (9), 1975–1985.

Pernille, B., Christensen, L.R., 2011. Relation work: creating socio-technical connections in global engineering, Paper presented at the ECSCW 2011 Proceedings of the 12th European Conference on Computer Supported Cooperative Work. Aarhus, Denmark, pp. 24–28 September.

Pinder, R., Petchey, R., Shaw, S., Carter, Y., 2005. What's in a care pathway? Towards a cultural cartography of the new NHS. Sociol. Health Illn. 27 (6), 759–779.

Smith, G.W., 2018. Paper Safe: The Triumph of Bureaucracy in Safety Management. Independently Published.

Strauss, A., Fagerhaugh, S., Suczet, B., Weiner, C., 1985. The Social Organization of Medical Work. University of Chicago Press, Chicago, IL.

Taylor, F.W., 1911. Principles of Scientific Management. Harper, New York.

Timmermans, S., Berg, M., 1997. Standardization in action: achieving local universality through medical protocols. Soc. Stud. Sci. 27 (2), 273–305.

Timmermans, S., Berg, M., 2003. The Gold Standard: The Challenge of Evidence-based Medicine and Standardization in Health Care. Temple University Press, Philadelphia, PA.

Waring, J.J., Bishop, S., 2010. Lean healthcare: rhetoric, ritual and resistance. Soc. Sci. Med. 71 (7), 1332–1340. doi:10.1016/j.socscimed.2010.06.028.

Weick, K.E., 1995. Sense-Making in Organizations. Sage, Thousand Oaks, CA.

Womack, J.P., Jones, D.T., 1996. Lean Thinking: Banish Waste and Create Wealth in Your Corporation. Simon & Schuster, Manhattan, New York City.

Suggested Reading

The Relationship Between Emergent and Rational–Linear Forms of Organisation

Checkland, K., Hammond, J., Allen, P., Coleman, A., Warwick-Giles, L., Hall, A., et al., 2019. Road to nowhere? A critical consideration of the use of the metaphor 'care pathway' in health services planning, organisation and delivery. J. Soc. Policy 49 (2), 405–424.

A critical exploration of the metaphor of a care pathway for commissioning and planning healthcare. Drawing on research on the reorganisation of the English National Health Service, the authors argue that the metaphor of a pathway suggests a limited range of approaches and solutions to service design which may make planning more difficult. They propose an alternative metaphor—the service map—and consider how service planning processes might be altered by using an alternative metaphor.

Mæhle, P.M., Hanto, I.K.S., Smeland, S., 2020. Practicing integrated care pathways in Norwegian hospitals: coordination through industrialized standardization, value chains, and quality management or an organizational equivalent to improvised jazz standards. Int. J. Environ. Res. Publ. Health 17 (24), 9199.

A qualitative study which examined the implementation of cancer care pathways in Norway and the challenges of using a standardised approach in conditions which call for emergent models.

Timmermans, S., Berg, M., 2003. The Gold Standard: The Challenge of Evidence-Based Medicine and Standardization in Healthcare. Temple University Press, Philadelphia, PA.

A classic book in science and technology studies, which cuts through the polarised debates on standards and standardization in healthcare, to explore both the risks and benefits to patients and healthcare professionals alike.

CHAPTER 5

Care Trajectory Management and Healthcare Quality and Safety

LEARNING OUTCOMES

At the end of this chapter, you will be able to:

- Explain the different ways in which poor coordination impacts on healthcare quality and safety
- Discuss the importance of care trajectory management for the quality and safety of patient care
- Describe and explain approaches to addressing the challenges of care coordination

Introduction

This chapter explores why care trajectory management matters for patients and the quality and safety of the care they receive. High-quality healthcare does not hinge on individual brilliance—as seductive as such portrayals might be—but on ensuring that all the elements required to support an individual's needs for care and treatment—the people, the materials, the technologies and the expertise—are assembled and aligned when they are needed (Baker et al., 2020; Stewart et al., 2021). 'Right care, right place, right time' may be the holy grail of healthcare quality and safety, but for the reasons outlined in earlier chapters, this is not easy to achieve. This chapter will examine evidence from a variety of healthcare contexts to consider the implications of poor coordination for the quality and safety of healthcare. It will also review how insights on organisational resilience informed by complexity science are stimulating fresh approaches to addressing this intractable challenge and consider the implications of these new ways of thinking for care trajectory management.

Care Coordination and Healthcare Quality and Safety: Patient Case Studies

This section centres on three patient case studies. Each focuses on an individual's care and treatment and the impacts of poor coordination on the quality and safety of their care. The first case—Julie Carman (Case Study 5.1)—features on Patient Stories, a web-based resource which uses

---

CASE STUDY 5.1   Julie Carman

In 2008, Julie Carman was involved in a road traffic accident whilst on a cycling holiday. She suffered injuries to her face, jaw and legs but made a good initial recovery and expected to return to work within 3 months.

Three *years* later she was still undergoing treatment having experienced two further emergency admissions to hospital due to acute cellulitis and sepsis. A series of 'everyday' communication failures conspired to create delays in her treatment. These led to a slower recovery and in Julie's view were very probably avoidable.

Everyone was very kind to me but no one did anything. A number of medical people said, 'Oh you'll feel better when you get some IV antibiotics', but no one actually gave me any [....] I would say that if they were evaluated individually, they would come out fine, but I kept falling through the gaps.

With permission from Anderson-Wallace, M. Julie's story. Patient Stories, 22 August 2023. http://www.patient-stories.org.uk/recent-posts/julies-story-now-available/ (Accessed 12 December 2022).

---

digital and media approaches to provoke debate about patient safety and patient's experiences of healthcare. Julie's story is summarised here, but the full account of her experiences can be accessed on the website (http://www.patientstories.org.uk/recent-posts/julies-story-now-available/). The coordination failure in Julie's case was relatively simple, but the impact on Julie's recovery was profound.

Julie's experience could have been very different if it were not for what she calls the 'everyday communication failures', which resulted in her not receiving vital antibiotics when needed. From Julie's perspective, it wasn't that individual providers were uncaring or incompetent; rather, her care fell through the gaps in the system.

Our second case was reported by the BBC and relates to a failure of communication between nurses and healthcare assistants (Case Study 5.2).

The reporting of this case is puzzling and leaves many questions unanswered. For example, coeliac disease does not usually cause vomiting, and thus, it is possible that the Weetabix may not have been the source of the sequence of events which led to the patient death. Following the inquest, however, the coroner was contacted by many members of the public who had read media coverage of the case to express concerns about the care of people with coeliac disease in hospital. In response, the coroner appointed an independent expert gastroenterologist to review the evidence, before concluding her report and determining whether a Prevention of Future Death (PFD) report was required (BBC, 2022) (Box 5.1). At the time of writing, the case had not been

---

CASE STUDY 5.2   Hazel Pearson

On 17 June 2022 Tom Ambrose reported on the findings of an inquest into the death of Hazel Pearson, an 80-year-old woman admitted with a pleural effusion to Wrexham Maelor Hospital in Flintshire, Wales. Hazel had coeliac disease, an autoimmune disorder, in which the body attacks its own tissues after consuming gluten, causing damage to the small intestine.

Hazel died in hospital with aspiration pneumonia within days of being fed Weetabix, a breakfast cereal containing gluten. The inquest heard that although her condition was noted in the admission documents, there was no sign at her bedside to indicate she had coeliac disease, which meant healthcare assistants were unaware of her dietary needs. Hazel became unwell and vomited shortly after eating her breakfast, and it was later found that she had aspirated stomach contents into her lungs.

The hospital matron informed the inquest that changes had been made following the incident, including placing signs above beds for patients with special dietary requirements. However, the assistant coroner criticised the plan as 'amateurish', indicating that there were further questions for the health board to answer before the report could be concluded. The inquest was adjourned.

Ambrose, T., 2022. Coeliac patient died days after being fed Weetabix, inquest hears. https://www.bbc.co.uk/news/uk-wales-61836866 (Accessed 12 December 2022).

BOX 5.1 ■ Definition: Prevention of Future Death Reports

In the UK coroners have a legal power and duty to write a report following an inquest if it appears that there is a risk of other deaths occurring in similar circumstances. Prevention of Future Death (PFD) reports are issued by coroners if they believe action should be taken to prevent a future death. Reports are sent to the people or organisations who can take action to reduce risk. They must reply within 56 days to say what action they plan to take.

---

concluded. For current purposes, however, feeding Weetabix to a patient with coeliac disease was an error, the result of a failure to communicate adequately Hazel's dietary requirements to the healthcare assistants responsible for assisting with eating. Was the coroner justified in describing the hospital's response as 'amateurish'? What other measures could be put in place to prevent this from happening in the future?

The final case study is derived from the experiences of George Brown (Case Study 5.3), a distant family member. The following description was crafted from a comprehensive letter of complaint sent to the hospital which catalogued a series of shortcomings in George's care. This example was first published in *The Invisible Work of Nurses* (Allen, 2015) and is used here with the consent of the family who requested that George should not remain anonymous in the hope that his experiences could be used to address service shortcomings for the benefit of others.

The case of George Brown illustrates the important role of the family in ensuring continuity of care, where communications between the different parts of the healthcare system were inadequate. Had it not been for the family's intervention, George's needs in relation to his recent surgery would have been overlooked.

Together, the case studies offer powerful illustrations of the consequences of poor coordination for patients and their families. Each case may be unique, but there is compelling evidence that failures of coordination form part of a wider pattern. Despite the invisible efforts of nurses, poor care coordination is a leading cause of failures in healthcare quality and safety with negative impacts on patient outcomes (Institute of Medicine, 2001; Leary et al., 2021; Tarrant et al., 2015) and the cost of care (Frandsen, 2015). The next part of this chapter reviews some of the research evidence in this area.

CASE STUDY 5.3 | George Brown

Following a diagnosis of bowel cancer George Brown was admitted to hospital for surgery on 9 January 2012 and underwent an 8-hour operation. Postoperatively he developed severe peritonitis and required admission to the Intensive Care Unit. Notwithstanding this complication, George eventually made a good recovery from his surgery and was able to be discharged home. On 28 February 2012 George was readmitted to hospital by his primary care doctor following an episode of breathlessness and light headedness. After spending some time in the Medical Assessment Unit, he was eventually admitted to the Coronary Care Unit with cardiac arrhythmias. After several days, in the light of George's conversations with members of his family, it became evident that the staff on the Coronary Care Unit had little information on George's previous surgery and consequently his nutritional and dietary requirements, all central to his postoperative recovery, had been overlooked. The family spoke to the nurse in Coronary Care Unit who managed to locate and supply George with the supplementary energy drinks that he had been previously prescribed and arranged for a nutritional assessment. This also precipitated the ward to organise meetings with the cardiac, surgical and oncology teams to discuss George's care.

With permission from Taylor & Francis Group. Allen, D. 2015. The Invisible Work of Nurses: Hospitals, Organisation and Healthcare. Routledge, London and New York. p. 108

Care Coordination and Healthcare Quality and Safety: A Review of Research Evidence

EVIDENCE FROM PREVENTION OF FUTURE DEATH REPORTS

Leary et al. (2021) reviewed PFD reports (see Box 5.1) from 2016 to 2019 for deaths in hospitals, care homes and community settings in England and Wales. A total of 710 reports were examined, with 3469 concerns being raised. After examining the structure and quality of the data, thematic analysis was undertaken. Thematic analysis is a form of pattern recognition in which themes derived from the data become the categories for analysis. The PFD reports were analysed by three researchers, and Cohen's kappa coefficient (κ) statistic was used to establish the degree of agreement between the researchers in categorising data. Fifty-three subcategories of concern were identified which were grouped into five themes indicating the overarching safety issue:

- a deficit in skill or knowledge
- missed, delayed or uncoordinated care
- communication and cultural issues
- system issues
- lack of resources

A major theme was missed, delayed or uncoordinated care, which included the following sub-themes: care, investigations and assessments that were not done or significantly delayed (this reso-nates with Case Study 5.1 in this chapter); uncoordinated or unmanaged care (this resonates with Case Study 5.3 in this chapter); absent or poor assessment of care needs; no or insufficient care plan (this resonates with Case Study 5.2); insufficient advice on self-care (this relates to the discussion in Chapter 3 on the work of patients); inappropriate care setting (this issue and its role in care trajectory management will be considered in subsequent chapters); and inappropriate or absent medications management (see Box 3.6, Chapter 3). Most cases in the PFD reports involved more than one issue.

The kind of analysis undertaken by Leary et al. offers valuable insights into the issues identified by coroners in their reports, themes, which the authors note mirror those identified in non-fatal error reporting (Aaronson et al., 2019). However, in the healthcare safety literature, a distinction is made between proximal and distal factors contributing to suboptimal care. Proximal factors indicate a close relationship to the issues, whereas a distal factor is more removed. If a root cause analysis of specific cases (Box 5.2) was carried out, it is quite possible that the organisation of care could have been a distal contributory factor in many of the other themes arising from Leary et al.'s report. Work through Exercise 5.1 to test this suggestion.

EVIDENCE FROM HOSPITAL CARE

Kobewka et al. (2016) carried out a hospital-wide review of mortality (Box 5.4) to understand the quality-of-care problems associated with patient deaths.

BOX 5.2 ▪ Definition: Root Cause Analysis

Root cause analysis is an approach used to learn from critical incidents. It is designed to identify system and process vulnerabilities rather than blaming individuals. It is informed by human factors engineering.

EXERCISE 5.1

Review the code book of subthemes identified by Leary et al. (2021) (Box 5.3). Considering what you have learnt about proximal and distal factors, select which categories of concern might be attrib-uted to failures of care coordination or organisation and note the reasoning behind your answer.

You can record your answer in the Care Trajectory Management Workbook (see Evolve website).

BOX 5.3 ■ Category of Prevention of Future Death Concerns Code Book Subthemes

Deficit in skill or expertise
Failure to deviate from algorithmic care or policy when harmful or inappropriate
Failure to be aware of, follow or implement evidence-based guidance
Misprescribing
Misdiagnosis
Unnecessary or inappropriate investigations or care
Inappropriate equipment usage
Human error during procedures
Care (including investigations and assessments) not done
Failure to report concerns to the organisational leaders or regulator
Reactive culture
Ergonomics and design of equipment
Equipment failure
IT unsuitability/failure
Failure to share records in IT platforms across organisations
Unable to access records (paper or IT)
Care (including investigations and assessments) significantly delayed
Uncoordinated/unmanaged care
No/poor assessment of care needs
No or insufficient care plan
No or insufficient advice on self-care
Inappropriate care setting (no or inadequate assessment)
No or inappropriate medicines management (polypharmacy/overprescribing/oversupply of medication)
Failure/refusal to communicate with other team members or agencies
Failure/refusal to communicate with carers/families
Poor/unsuitable environment
Contracting or financial disputes
Failure to provide care/treatment due to demand management policy/strategy
Reorganisation of services
No or insufficient learning form internal investigations
Concerns about postmortem procedures
Medicines unavailability
Out-of-date applications ('apps')
Failure to document care
Retrospective documentation both after the fact (question of reliability) or with alleged intent to deceive
Language or cultural misunderstanding
Inconsistent terminology
Missing notes/documents
Staff stress
Refusal to treat
Dishonesty
Failure or absent leadership
Misuse of equipment
Inappropriate use of resources (i.e., police)
Lack of policy/guidance
Regulatory issues
Untraceable staff
No response to coroner
Equipment missing
No or insufficient staffing
High workloads
Unable to recruit
Lack of staffed beds

IT, Information technology.
From Leary, A., Bushe, D., Oldman, C., Lawler, J., Punshon, G., 2021. A thematic analysis of the Prevention of Future Deaths reports in healthcare from HM coroners in England and Wales 2016–2019. J. Patient Saf. Risk Manag. 26(1), 14–21. doi:10.1177/2516043521992651.

A nurse and a physician independently reviewed every death that occurred over a 3-month period in a Canadian teaching hospital. They identified deaths that were unanticipated, or where the experience offered an opportunity to learn from the case to improve care delivery. These cases were reviewed by a multidisciplinary committee. A total of 427 deaths were reviewed in detail; 33 (7.7%) deaths were considered unanticipated, and 100 (23.4%) deaths were judged to be associated with the possibility of improvement in care delivery. Table 5.1 summarises the occurrence of different improvement opportunities identified in the study.

The most common gap in care, accounting for over 25% of those opportunities for improvement identified, was 'goals of care not discussed, or the discussion was inadequate' and clearly a case of poor coordination. As with the earlier example, a root cause analysis of specific cases, taking both distal and proximal factors into account, would likely identify that the organisation of care could have been a distal contributory factor in almost all the opportunities for improvement listed by the authors. For example, delays in surgery may arise because of the omission of an essential

---

BOX 5.4 ■ Definition: Hospital Mortality

Hospital mortality refers to patients who died during or shortly after admission to hospital (Goodacre et al., 2015).

Goodacre, S., Campbell, M., Carter, A., 2015. What do hospital mortality rates tell us about quality of care? Emerg. Med. J. 32(3), 244–247. doi:10.1136/emermed-2013-203022.

TABLE 5.1 ■ Opportunities for Improvement as Classified by the Corporate Mortality-Review Committee

Opportunity for Improvement	Number of Occurrences (N = 97)
Goals of care were not discussed, or the discussion was inadequate	25
Delay in diagnosis or failure to achieve a diagnosis	8
Uncontrolled pain	7
Inappropriate delay in transfer to hospice or long-term care	7
Developed a pressure ulcer in hospital	5
Did not receive a treatment that was indicated	5
Appropriate specialists were not involved in the patient's care	5
Fall in hospital	4
Delay in surgery that affected patient's outcome and contributed to death	4
Hospital-acquired infection	3
Had multiple ER visits leading to admission and did not receive appropriate treatment	3
Complications of a procedure	2
Admission to hospital was unnecessary. There was no care given in hospital that the patient was not already receiving at their place of residence	2
Inadequate assessment and consideration of preoperative risk	2
Inadequate monitoring of an unstable patient	2
Error made during surgery	2
Other	11

ER, Emergency room.

Reproduced with permission from Kobewka, D., van Walraven, C., Turnball, J., Worthington, J., Calder, L., Forster, A., 2016. Quality gaps identified through mortality review. BMJ Qual. Saf. 26, 141–149.

preoperative activity; inadequate monitoring may have been owing to a failure of intershift handover; and uncontrolled pain could occur if junior doctors are unavailable to prescribe medications.

EVIDENCE FROM TRANSITIONS OF CARE

While poor coordination *within* care settings can have a negative impact on healthcare quality and safety, the problem is particularly acute when patients transition across departmental and organisational boundaries. For example, studies show that the quality of care can be suboptimal during, or because of, hospital discharge (Laugaland et al., 2012). Data provided by the former English National Patient Safety Agency (2009) indicate that 'transfer/discharge of patient and infrastructure' accounted for 7%–8% of reported safety incidents in 2009, with 'notifying and organising external services' identified as the most common category of reported incident. These figures probably underestimate the scale of the problem because most incident reporting systems are not well utilised across health and social care boundaries (Waring et al., 2016).

Waring et al. (2016) carried out a large-scale qualitative study to explore patient safety at hospital discharge in stroke and hip fracture patients in the English National Health Service. The transition from hospital to home in these two patient groups often involves complex arrangements and the organisation and coordination of multiple health and social care providers. The study involved narrative interviews with 213 stakeholders and professionals involved in discharge planning and care transition activities. Narrative interviews invite participants to summarise their experiences of an event and tell their stories to the interviewer. Participants in the study were asked about their experiences of discharge planning processes, examples of unsafe discharges and their perceptions about the sources of safety or risk and how discharge planning processes might be improved. Narratives were analysed in line with 'systems' thinking to identity the factors involved in threats to safety. As described in Chapter 4, systems thinking understands phenomenon as part of a wider interconnected whole in which different components interact with each other. Four common safety incidents were identified from participants' accounts: falls; medications management; infection, sores and ulceration; and relapse (Table 5.2).

TABLE 5.2 ■ Summary of Safety Incidents Identified by Waring et al. (2016)

Safety Issue	Description
Falls	Falls at home or in the care setting after discharge from hospital
	Falls that occurred as the patient was in transit from hospital to the discharge destination
	Falls occurring on the ward after a delayed discharge, possibly because of lower levels of supervision from staff and higher aspirations for independence on the part of the patient
Medicines management	Problems with medicines reconciliation between hospital and primary care doctors, for example, poor communication about changes to normal medications
	Problems with medicines adherence at discharge, owing to poor education, administration difficulties, cognitive problems
	Medicines dispensing errors
Infection, ulceration or sores	Community staff identified that there was an issue with patients being discharged home with unhealed pressure ulcers or infections which could be better managed in hospital
	Infections, ulcers or sores could also develop in the community after discharge
Relapse	Concerns expressed about premature discharge from hospital without the appropriate community support arrangements

Waring, J., Bishop, S., Marshall, F., 2016. A qualitative study of professional and carer perceptions of the threats to safe hospital discharge for stroke and hip fracture patients in the English National Health Service. BMC Health Serv. Res. 14(16), 297.

Waring et al. (2016) identified proximal and distal factors that participants described as contributing to safety incidents (Table 5.3).

In discussing their findings, Waring et al. highlight how little the study participants understood about the system factors that contributed to safety threats and how their accounts were characterised by a tendency to allocate responsibilities for failures to other actors. Social care professionals found fault with hospital staff and primary care doctors, ward nurses and therapists criticised medical decision making. This is a good example of the challenges of coordination created by the distributed nature of healthcare work and the partial understanding of the overall trajectory of care that this produces (see Chapter 3, Complexity 3: Healthcare Is Distributed Work). Before reading further, work through Exercise 5.2.

It was difficult for community social care providers to describe in detail why equipment might be missing, but they would infer or assume it was related to either the equipment supply or ordering processes. Similarly, those in the hospital environment had limited appreciation of the safety events that transpired in the community, such as the significance of an undiagnosed infection or ulcer. In other words, participants' understanding of discharge safety was shaped by their distinct position within the care process and the 'sight-line' or scope of perception this afforded for understanding either the preceding causes of an event, or the consequences of their actions.

Waring et al. (2016, p. 11)

EXERCISE 5.2

Review the proximal and distal factors contributing to safety threats during hospital discharge identified by Waring et al. (2016) (Table 5.3) and identify the safety threats at discharge in which the coordination or organisation of care was *not* a contributory factor. Explain the reasons for your answers. You can record your answer in the Care Trajectory Management Workbook (see Evolve website).

TABLE 5.3 ■ **Proximal and Distal Factors Contributing to Safety Issues During Hospital Discharge in Stroke and Hip Fracture Patients Identified by Waring et al. (2016)**

Category of Threat	Examples	Explanation
Proximal 'contributing' factors Definition: actions, conditions or triggers that were seen as the primary or immediate cause of a safety incident	Assessment of patient	This refers to disagreements between the team as to whether the patient is ready for discharge, and uncertainty about whether medical fitness was a sufficient basis on which to progress a discharge. Other issues related to the failure of the acute sector to address secondary health problems, which could be consequential for the success of discharge plans.
	Completion of tests	Participants described that some tests ordered during discharge planning were not completed. Some patients were discharged before tests results were back.
	Ordering and use of equipment	Bureaucratic processes for ordering. Uncertain lines of responsibility across health and social care providers. Delays in equipment installation. Poor education of patients and families on equipment use. Different technologies used in hospital and community context.
	Provision and management of medicines	The prescriptions of medications to take home were rushed, inaccurate or incomplete. Inadequate checking of medications before discharge. Patients and families reported poor information on medication management.

Category of Threat	Examples	Explanation
	Follow-up care and monitoring	Hospital participants highlighted issues arising from inadequate support provided in the community, including the limited involvement of the primary care doctor following discharge from hospital.
Distal latent factors Definition: distal factors included those underlying or system-level issues that participants commonly described while explaining why a safety event might have occurred and which were understood as an enduring or cross-cutting issue that impacted upon care quality through shaping the context in which more proximal factors occurred.	Discharge planning	There was no standardised process for discharge planning and 'a general sense of complexity, confusion and poor integration between the different health and social are systems of work that was seen as conditioning many of the problems of care planning'. There were challenges in involving all team members in planning meetings; 'this meant that concerns about patient mobility, cognition or lifestyle factors were not fully considered […] [and] on-going discharge plans would often be incomplete or missing important detail'.
	Referral processes	Many problems were associated with referral processes to community and social services. Paperwork associated with referral processes was perceived to be excessive. Accessing patient information to make a referral was difficult when information was spread across multiple record keeping systems.
	Discharge timing	Participants highlighted the problem of premature discharge on the one hand, and delayed discharge on the other. It could be difficult to agree the timing of discharge with the work schedules of acute and community providers.
	Resource constraints	Participants highlighted the challenges of constraints on community resources which could delay discharge or create the conditions in which discharge arrangements were suboptimal.
	Organisational demands	Participants pointed to the pressures on acute hospital beds and patient flow and the constraints on the availability of social care provision in the community.

Waring, J., Bishop, S., Marshall, F., 2016. A qualitative study of professional and carer perceptions of the threats to safe hospital discharge for stroke and hip fracture patients in the English National Health Service. BMC Health Serv. Res. 14(16), 297.

EVIDENCE FROM PLANNED CARE

This final example in this section concerns coordination in scheduled surgery. Weinberg et al. (2007) investigated individuals' experience of coordination in their postoperative care in 222 patients who had undergone elective unilateral knee replacement in a North American healthcare organisation. Treatment was undertaken in the acute hospital and then continued in a rehabilitation facility. Data were generated through a survey instrument, administered before surgery and at 6 and 12 weeks postoperatively. Patient outcomes used in the study were postoperative pain and functional status, measured through 17 items from the Western Ontario and McMaster University Osteoarthritis Index (WOMAC). WOMAC is a validated questionnaire completed by patients which assesses clinical outcomes with knee or hip osteoarthritis (Bellamy et al., 1988). Patients' experience of coordination as they transitioned between settings was measured using items from the Picker Post-Acute Care Survey for joint patients (The Picker Institute, 2006). These items addressed two aspects of continuity: informational continuity—providers and patients having the information they need—and management continuity—providers showing agreement about care and patients knowing the next steps.

The study found that patients reported problems with coordination between the hospital and rehabilitation settings and between providers and themselves. Coordination between patients and providers created the most problems for patients, whether coordination for discharge or communication of information relevant for patients' treatment. Many reported not having the information

EXERCISE 5.3

'Failing to provide professional coordination and leaving coordination solely to patients and their caregivers signals a dysfunctional system' (Stille et al., 2005). To what extent do you agree/disagree with this assertion? Document the reasons for your answer.

You can record your answer in the Care Trajectory Management Workbook (see Evolve website).

needed to manage their condition after their return home. Patients' reports also highlighted coordination breakdowns between providers. Not only did patients report problems in the way that staff worked together, but they also reported problems related to transitions between settings, with receiving providers not having important information about patients' history, surgery or special needs or conditions. These were more than minor irritations about the service. These problems, measured at 6 weeks after surgery, were associated with greater joint pain, lower functioning and lower patient satisfaction. At 12 weeks after surgery, coordination problems were associated with greater joint pain, but were not associated with functional status.

Elective surgery is an area of healthcare where routines and standards have a central role in coordinating care. It is a planned procedure, patients are preoptimised for surgery, and it is a high-volume activity. Care trajectory management should be relatively straightforward, compared with the hip fracture and stroke patients in Waring et al.'s (2016) study considered in the previous section. Commenting on their findings, the authors express surprise that these failures of coordination should occur in very standardised, planned and predictable care processes which should be amenable to rational-linear models of organisation:

> *These findings are striking because they were obtained in connection with a highly routine, elective procedure with a high rate of patient satisfaction and success in improving pain and functioning. Even within this successful scenario, improvements in coordination made significant improvement in clinical outcomes.*
>
> Weinberg et al. (2007, p. 20)

The surgeons involved identified time, patient volume and the inability to access other providers as a key barrier to coordination. These barriers were the consequences of market mechanisms which had prompted surgeons and others to increase their caseloads and had reduced their time available for coordinating care for each patient. A consequence of this was an increased need for patients to coordinate their own care, adding to the significant illness burden that users and caregivers already face (see Box 3.2, Chapter 3). It is possible to envisage similar impacts in publicly funded healthcare systems, where waiting list targets or resource restrictions produce comparable constraints. Before reading further, work through Exercise 5.3.

Addressing the Challenges of Care Coordination

In the face of mounting evidence of the relationship between coordination and healthcare quality and safety, it is not surprising that effecting improvements in this area is an international policy priority. For example, a World Health Organization Europe (2012) report maintained that service fragmentation and insufficient coherence are the main factors inhibiting the efficiency of interventions and the quality of healthcare outcomes. In the North American context, the Lucian Leape Institute report *Order From Chaos: Accelerating Care Integration* (Lucian Leape Institute, 2012) concluded that poor care integration is linked to adverse events, and should be among the top priorities for achieving consistently safe, effective and efficient healthcare. These observations are echoed in several major national reviews of patient safety (Institute of Medicine, 2001; National Patient Safety Agency, 2007; The Health Foundation, 2011).

In the wake of such calls to action, wide-ranging initiatives to improve the organisation and integration of care have been implemented across the industrialised world. Processes and structures have been reengineered (Agency for Healthcare Research and Quality, 2013; Morris et al., 2014); a raft of coordinating technologies—care pathways, protocols and algorithms—have been developed (Allen, 2009); specialist coordinator roles have emerged (McMurray and Cooper, 2016); interventions to improve hospital discharge have been implemented (Gandhi et al., 2018); and a range of financial incentives deployed (Zutshi et al., 2014). But despite several decades of activity, improvements in care coordination have only been incremental (Gandhi et al., 2018) and progress has remained elusive (Braithwaite, 2018).

Drawing on insights from complexity science and resilience engineering (Hollnagel et al., 2006), a growing number of leaders in this field are calling for a changed mindset in understanding healthcare for the purposes of improvement (Braithwaite, 2018; Greenhalgh and Papoutsi, 2018; Penprase and Norris, 2005).

In the past, healthcare improvement efforts have been based on an idealised view of how activities are performed, with interventions designed to bring work-as-done more in alignment with work-as-imagined. The popularity of this approach can be traced back to the success of scientific management theory, introduced by Frederick Taylor at the beginning of the 20th century (see Chapter 4, Rational–Linear Organisation). Taylor demonstrated how breaking a complex activity into discrete tasks could improve work efficiency, culminating in the establishment of the factory production line. However, in complex systems of work, such as healthcare, task performance needs to be continuously adjusted to match the changing conditions, such that work-as-done differs significantly from work-as-imagined. Proponents of a complexity science approach argue that improvement efforts should start by paying more attention to how care is delivered at the frontline, to really understand real-life work processes. Additionally, they argue, instead of only focusing on when things go wrong (root cause analyses and adverse event reporting), advances in healthcare improvement will come from attending to when things go right, and better understanding how complex systems function, despite their instability and unpredictability. Within complexity science, there is a growing interest in understanding how everyday practices, and the continued adjustments made by healthcare practitioners, provide healthcare systems with their *resilience* (Box 5.5); that is, they enable the organisation to function despite the unpredictable qualities of the work. From this perspective, then, the most powerful processes begin with the staff and their interventions in responding to contingencies in the work environment (Penprase and Norris, 2005). It is in this context that formal acknowledgement of the nursing contribution to the organisation and coordination of care is long overdue.

BOX 5.5 ■ Improving Organisational Resilience in Healthcare

In response to the very real challenges of bringing about improvements in healthcare quality and safety, researchers are starting to apply insights from resilience engineering to healthcare systems (Hollnagel et al., 2006). Resilience engineering was put forward as a framework for thinking about safety as a complement to established approaches to industrial safety. As the approach has evolved in its application across several fields—air traffic control, nuclear power generation, offshore production, commercial fishing—resilience has come to be understood as the intrinsic quality of a system to adjust its functioning prior to, during or following changes and disruptions, so that it can maintain its operation in expected and unexpected circumstances. Resilience is not so much a quality that a system has, rather it is a characteristic of how it functions—that is, what it does.

Hollnagel, E., Woods, D.D., Leveson, N. (Eds.), 2006. Resilience Engineering: Concepts and Precepts. Ashgate, Aldershot, UK.

Summary

This chapter examined the relationship between care coordination and the quality and safety of patient care. It considered three case studies of the real-life impacts of coordination failures and then reviewed in detail some examples from the research evidence. While improving care coordination has been an international healthcare priority for several decades, it is proving to be an intractable problem. The chapter concluded by introducing alternative approaches to addressing service improvement informed by complexity science, based on an understanding of the work as it is done, rather than as it is imagined, to better understand how the actions of staff contribute to organisational resilience. It is in this context that care trajectory management demands to be formally recognised in policy and practice.

SUMMARY OF KEY LEARNING

- There is strong research evidence that failures of coordination have negative impacts on the quality and safety of patient care.
- This is a recurrent pattern across international healthcare contexts.
- This picture remains largely unaltered despite decades of interventions intended to address these challenges.
- Leaders in complexity science have made the case for rethinking how we approach these challenges, by focusing on the work as it is done, and better understanding why things go right rather than simply concentrating on when things go wrong.
- Care trajectory management makes an important contribution to the coordination of care in healthcare systems by constituting an invisible safety net which contributes to organisational resilience.

QUICK QUIZ

- What is a Prevention of Future Deaths report?
- What is the difference between proximal and distal factors in understanding service processes?
- What is root cause analysis?
- What is resilience engineering?
- What is organisational resilience?

References

Aaronson, E.L., Brown, D., Benzer, T., Natsui, S., Mort, E., 2019. Incident reporting in emergency medicine: a thematic analysis of events. J. Patient Saf. 15, e60–e63.

Agency for Healthcare Research and Quality, 2013. Re-engineered Discharge (RED) Toolkit: Tool 1 Overview. Agency for Healthcare Research and Quality, Rockville, MD.

Allen, D., 2009. From boundary concept to boundary object: the politics and practices of care pathway development. Soc. Sci. Med. 69 (3), 354–361.

Allen, D., 2015. The Invisible Work of Nurses: Hospitals, Organisation and Healthcare. Routledge, London and New York.

Baker, R., Freeman, G.K., Haggerty, J.L., Bankart, M.J., Nockels, K.H., 2020. Primary medical care continuity and patient mortality: a systematic review. Br. J. Gen. Pract. 70 (698), e600–e611. doi:10.3399/bjgp20X712289.

BBC, 2022. Coeliac patient death: expert to review inquest evidence. https://www.bbc.co.uk/news/uk-wales-62822094 (Accessed 12 December 2022).

Bellamy, N., Buchanan, W.W., Goldsmith, C.H., Campbell, J., Stitt, L.W., 1988. Validation study of WOMAC: a health status instrument for measuring clinically important patient relevant outcomes to antirheumatic drug therapy in patients with osteoarthritis of the hip or knee. J. Rheumatol. 15, 1833–1840.

Braithwaite, J., 2018. Changing how we think about healthcare improvement. Br. Med. J. 361, 1–5.

Frandsen, B.R., Joynt, K.E., Rebitzer, J.B., Jha, A.K., 2015. Care fragmentation, quality, and costs among chronically ill patients. Am. J. Manag. Care. 21 (5), 355–362.

Gandhi, T., Kaplan, G., Leape, L., Berwick, D., Edgman-Levitan, S., Edmondon, A., et al., 2018. Transforming concepts in patient safety: a progress report. BMJ Qual. Saf. 27, 1019–1026. doi:10.1136/bmjqs-2017-007756.

Greenhalgh, T., Papoutsi, C., 2018. Studying complexity in health services research: desperately seeking an overdue paradigm shift. BMC Med. 16 (95). doi:10.1186/s12916-018-1089-4.

Hollnagel, E., Woods, D.D., Leveson, N. (Eds.), 2006. Resilience Engineering: Concepts and Precepts. Ashgate, Aldershot, UK.

Institute of Medicine, 2001. Crossing the Quality Chasm: A New Health System for the 21st Century. Institute of Medicine, Washington, DC.

Kobewka, D., van Walraven, C., Turnball, J., Worthington, J., Calder, L., Forster, A., 2016. Quality gaps identified through mortality review. BMJ Qual. Saf. 26, 141–149.

Laugaland, K., Aase, K., Barach, P., 2012. Interventions to improve patient safety in transitional care – a review of the evidence. Work 41 (Suppl. 1), 2915–2924. doi:10.3233/WOR-2012-0544-2915.

Leary, A., Bushe, D., Oldman, C., Lawler, J., Punshon, G., 2021. A thematic analysis of the Prevention of Future Deaths reports in healthcare from HM coroners in England and Wales 2016–2019. J. Patient Saf. Risk Manag. 26 (1), 14–21. doi:10.1177/2516043521992651.

Lucian Leape Institute, 2012. Order from Chaos: Accelerating Care Integration. National Patient Safety Foundation, Boston, MA.

McMurray, A., Cooper, H., 2016. The nurse navigator: an evolving model of care. Collegian Aust. J. Nurs. Pract. Scholarsh. Res. 24 (2), 205–212.

Morris, S., Hunter, R., Ramsay, A., Boaden, R., McKevitt, C., Perry, C., et al., 2014. Impact of centralising acute stroke services in English metropolitan areas on mortality and length of stay: difference-in-differences analysis. Br. Med. J., 349, g4757.

National Patient Safety Agency, 2007. The Fifth Report from the Patient Safety Observatory. Safer Care for the Acutely Ill Patient: Learning From Serious Incidents. National Patient Safety Agency, London.

National Patient Safety Agency, 2009. National Reporting and Learning System Quarterly Data Summary – England. TSO, London.

Penprase, B., Norris, D., 2005. What nurse leaders should know about complex adaptive systems theory. Nurs. Leadersh. Forum. 9 (3), 127–132.

Stewart, I., Leary, A., Khakwani, A., Borthwick, D., Tod, A., Hubbard, R., et al., 2021. Do working practices of cancer nurse specialists improve clinical outcomes? Retrospective cohort analysis from the English National Lung Cancer Audit. Int. J. Nurs. Stud. 118, 103718. doi:10.1016/j.ijnurstu.2020.103718.

Stille, C.J., Jerant, A., Bell, D., Meltzer, D., Elmore, J.G., 2005. Coordinating care across diseases, settings, and clinicians: a key role for the generalist in practice. Ann. Intern. Med. 142, 700–708.

Tarrant, C., Windridge, K., Baker, R., Freeman, G., Boulton, M., 2015. 'Falling through gaps': primary care patients' accounts of breakdowns in experienced continuity of care. Fam. Pract. 32 (1), 82–87. doi:10.1093/fampra/cmu077.

The Health Foundation, 2011. Evidence Scan: Levels of Harm. The Health Foundation, London. https://www.health.org.uk/sites/default/files/LevelsOfHarm_0.pdf (Accessed 22 January 2022).

The Picker Institute, 2006. The Picker Survey. www.picker.org.

Waring, J., Bishop, S., Marshall, F., 2016. A qualitative study of professional and carer perceptions of the threats to safe hospital discharge for stroke and hip fracture patients in the English National Health Service. BMC Health Serv. Res. 14 (16), 297.

Weinberg, D., Gittell, J., Lusenhop, R., Kautz, C., Wright, J., 2007. Beyond our walls: impact of patient and provider coordination across the continuum of outcomes for surgical patients. Health Serv. Res. 42, 7–24.

World Health Organization Europe, 2012. Modern Health Care Delivery Systems: Care Coordination and the Role of Hospitals. World Health Organization Europe, Copenhagen, Denmark.

Zutshi, A., Peikes, D., Smith, K., 2014. The Medical Home: What Do We Know, What Do We Need to Know? Agency for Healthcare Research and Quality, Rockville, MD.

Suggested Reading

Healthcare Quality and Safety

Aase, K., Waring, J., Schibevaag, L. (Eds.), 2017. Researching Quality in Care Transitions: International Perspectives. Palgrave Macmillan, Switzerland.

Allen, D., Braithwaite, G., Sandal, J., Waring, J. (Eds.), 2016. The Sociology of Healthcare Safety and Quality. Wiley Blackwell, Oxford.

Two edited collections of papers reporting research on healthcare quality and safety.

Complexity Science and Nursing

Penprase, B., Norris, D., 2005. What nurse leaders should know about complex adaptive systems theory. Nurs. Leadersh. Forum. 9 (3), 127–132.

An overview of key concepts in understanding complex adaptive systems theory and its application to nursing management. It highlights how thinking through complexity science calls for new ways of thinking and approaches to problem solving. It considers the contribution of self-organisation, to enable order and creativity to emerge, from the practices and creativity of staff.

CHAPTER 6

Care Trajectory Management and Professional Identity

LEARNING OUTCOMES

At the end of this chapter, you will be able to:
- Explain the invisibility of care trajectory management in nursing work
- Describe the consequences of care trajectory management's invisibility for nursing
- Explain the importance of care trajectory management for professional practice

Introduction

The previous chapter examined the relationship between care coordination and the quality and safety of healthcare and underlined the need to better understand how staff respond to everyday contingencies in the workplace to address this intractable problem. Having established why care trajectory management matters for patients, and why understanding the work-as-done is important to bring about improvements, this chapter considers the reasons for, and the professional and practical consequences of, the invisibility of care trajectory management work.

Why Is Care Trajectory Management Invisible Work?

If care trajectory management is so important for the quality and safety of patient care, why is it not a formally recognised element of the nursing role? Why is it invisible? No work is intrinsically visible or invisible. Work can be rendered invisible in different ways. Some work can be done in invisible places, such as the behind-the-screens body work of nurses (Lawler, 1991) and the backstage work of librarians (Nardi and Engeström, 1999). Work can also be done by invisible people. Hart (1991), who worked as a hospital domestic to study and experience this occupational role, notes how her visibility and invisibility within the organisation was socially structured.

I noticed that caterers – one step up from domestics – generally ignored me, while porters chatted and joked, I was invisible to doctors – particularly when mopping the stairs – while patients' visitors sought me out to ask directions.

Hart (1991, p. 85)

Care trajectory management is an example of functionally invisible work. Here the worker is visible, but the work is relegated to the background. If you look, you can see the work being done, but its taken-for-granted status means that it is invisible (Star and Strauss, 1999). So how has nursing arrived at this situation?

The answer to this question lies in the history of nursing's occupational development as a recognised profession. The late 19th and early 20th centuries saw a dramatic expansion of professions as we know them today (Perkin, 1989), and having established itself as a formal occupation, nursing, like many others, embarked on a process of professionalisation. Professionalisation refers to the activities through which an occupation seeks to secure legitimacy through the development of skills, identities and norms associated with the traits of a recognised profession (Box 6.1). A central quality of a profession is the claim to expert knowledge. Professions *profess* (Hughes, 1984); they profess to have exclusive expertise in a crucial aspect of life, and this is used to seek status and rewards for members. Abbott (1988) coined the term 'jurisdiction' to refer to the field of practice that forms the basis of a profession's knowledge claims. Professional status is not fixed; occupations exist in a system of work and are engaged in a process of creating, enforcing or fighting over jurisdictional boundaries in response to changes in the wider society (see Chapter 3, Box 3.3). The periodic boundary disputes among nursing, medicine and support staff are examples of these kinds of jurisdictional contests (Allen, 2001). It is through these processes established professions evolve, new professions emerge and some may disappear.

Nursing is a large and diverse profession which extends across different patient populations, specialisms and healthcare contexts. Compare, for example, the everyday work of a community mental health nurse with that of a nurse working in a day surgery unit, or a learning disability nurse working in a special school. Consider the knowledge and skills required by a critical care nurse, a paediatric oncology nurse or a homeless health nurse. The profession of nursing covers an unquestionably vast territory. While this makes for a rich array of career opportunities, it creates very real challenges for a professionalisation project. A major difficulty for nursing leaders has been to find a single unifying identity that encompasses the wide range of activities that comprise nursing work and which can be used as the basis for communicating the profession's claims to jurisdiction.

Nursing's early occupational development was characterised by an extraordinarily flexible scope of practice (Carpenter, 1977). The profession willingly embraced a broad range of work tasks, and consequently, by the 1960s the content of nursing work had expanded significantly. Advances in medical science had precipitated the delegation of new clinical responsibilities.

BOX 6.1 ■ Trait Models of Professionalism

Trait models of professionalism involved drawing up a list of criteria of a profession against which various occupations could be assessed (Greenwood, 1957). Relevant traits differentiated professions from nonprofessions and included possession and use of expert or specialist knowledge, exercise of autonomous thought and judgement, an ethical code and responsibility to wider society through voluntaristic commitment to a set of principles (Hoyle and John, 1995). While the trait model has been largely discredited in social science, it has nevertheless acted as a useful reference point by which occupations aspiring to professional status have sought to strengthen their social standing, through the acquisition of attributes taken to be signifiers of a true profession.

Greenwood, E., 1957. Attributes of a profession. Soc. Work. 2, 45–55.
Hoyle, E., John, P., 1995. Professional Knowledge and Professional Practice. Cassell, London.

There was an increase in the role of the nurse as the manager of a range of ancillary functions (such as cleaning and catering). Nursing work was also impacted by the growth in the number of people with long-term conditions. In the developed world, the 1960s and 1970s were characterised by a general belief in the efficacy of management techniques, and for a short period, it looked as if it was the management, rather than the clinical components of the nursing role, that was to be placed at the centre of nursing's professionalising strategy. In the UK, for example, the Salmon reforms aimed to modernise nursing management and extended the management chain above and below that of the matron. But while the reforms of nursing management advanced the interests of the nursing elite, they precipitated a progressive dilution of the wider nursing workforce and did nothing to address the dominance of medicine in the clinical sphere (Dingwall et al., 1988). The result was a period of professional unrest and a decisive reframing of nursing's professionalisation strategy, in which nursing's claim to jurisdiction was expressed almost exclusively in terms of its care-giving functions. This approach was driven in part by the influence of North American academic nurses, oriented to a trait model of professionalism, and committed to establishing a domain of practice that was autonomous from medicine, with an underpinning independent knowledge base. Appeals to 'care' differentiated nursing from the curative mandate of medicine and furnished nursing with an indefeasible argument with which to advance the interests of the profession; after all, who could be against 'care'?

Today, then, nursing is typically understood, and understands itself, as a care-giving profession (Allen, 2015). Informed by a distinctive holistic approach, models of nursing situate therapeutic relationships with patients and their families as the cornerstone of nursing practice (Allen, 2001; Armstrong, 1983; May, 1992). Indeed, nursing is widely regarded as *the* caring profession, and nursing is often referred to as a 'caring science' (Nelson and Gordon, 2006). But while nurses have mobilised around a collective professional identity centred on patient care, this framing has not been without tensions.

Across the world, nursing has faced continual challenges to justify its worth and has experienced a long history of persistent under funding. The precarious state of the global nursing workforce has been made even worse by the COVID-19 pandemic (Buchan et al., 2022). A wealth of empirical research highlights the mismatch between the work that nurses do and the predominant professional image (Box 6.2). Nurses are not only increasingly distant from direct care (Cavendish, 2013), but also they undertake a wide range of safety critical activities not captured by the prevailing professional image (Allen, 2004; Gordon and Nelson, 2006; Weinberg, 2006).

In a context in which nursing jurisdiction and practitioner identity have centred exclusively on nurse–patient relationships, the organisational component of nursing work has tended to be treated as the 'dirty work' of the profession (Hughes, 1984) (Box 6.3), at best an adjunct to the core nursing function, and at worse a distraction from the caring components of the nursing role. For example, the sociologist Celia Davies (1995) described nurses' 'professional predicament' in terms of the 'polo mint problem'. The polo mint is a sweet characterised by a hole at its centre, and the analogy is intended to signify the effect created by all the tasks required to support the healthcare system which, according to Davies, draw nurses away from patients and create a gap through which the caregiving function is lost. In a similar vein, a major preoccupation in studies of nursing work has been with the discrepancy between the primacy of nurses' caring role and the reality of everyday practice, and the measures that are necessary to return nurses to their rightful functions at the bedside (Hendrich et al., 2008; Hendrickson et al., 1990; Hollingsworth et al., 1998; Westbrook et al., 2011). (For another illustration, revisit the discussion of bureaucracy in Chapter 1: A Short History of the Organisational Component of Nursing Work).

Viewing nursing work through the prism of care trajectory management offers a different perspective. Rather than lamenting the dilution of caring, attention is focused on the network of activities that are involved in the organisational component of nursing and the circumstances that make these necessary. Given what we know about the unpredictable qualities of healthcare work,

BOX 6.2 ■ Disconnecting Care From Nursing Practice

A profession's claim to jurisdiction has implications for the professional identity of practitioners. It shapes how nurses think and talk about their work. Suzanne Gordon (2006), a journalist who has studied nursing, describes how by focusing on holism, nurses disconnect from their technical and medical expertise. She describes her experiences of talking about practice to a cohort of nurses returning to education to obtain a nurse practitioner degree. Nurse practitioners (NPs) have an advanced education and clinical skills, and work with an extended scope of practice, which overlaps with that of physicians. Gordon writes: 'When I asked the students to describe the work of the NP, all of them talked about the "holistic" approach of the nurse practitioner. In their discussion of "holism," they focused exclusively on psychosocial and emotional aspects of care. When I asked them about their medical knowledge of diseases and drugs, they seemed almost angry. "We take a holistic approach," one reiterated. When I suggested that holism includes the medical, she became distressed, insisting over and over again on "holism". Baffled by this response, I asked, "Doesn't holism include knowledge of routine medical conditions and your ability to diagnose them as well as to prescribe routine medical treatments? After all, don't nurse practitioners differ from the bedside nurse because they are legally permitted to diagnose routine conditions and prescribe medications? Wouldn't it be good to mention that?" I suggested.

Apparently not. This particular student felt that any mention of the medical would take away from the "nursing approach" and compromise the claim to holism. Another nurse [...] agreed. She seemed distraught by the idea that nurses would want to advertise their medical knowledge. To do so, she insisted, would be to "downplay" the holistic or psychosocial. Although I repeatedly insisted that I wanted the students to combine – not counterpose – it seemed difficult for them to capture that concept. "We have been trying to define our work with no success ever since I have been in nursing", the RN said in an agitated tone. "Trying to find something that is our own that no one can take away from us. Finally we have it. The NP role. We are the patient's partner, we give holistic care. We are patient-centred. And you are trying to take that away from us"' (Gordon, 2006, p. 115).

In another example, Dana Beth Weinberg (2006) studied the impacts on nurses of restructuring processes at Beth Israel Deaconess Medical Centre in 1999. A sociologist, with no background in nursing, Weinberg had only vague notions about nursing work, and throughout her study was repeatedly required to ask the question, 'What do nurses do?'. She writes that despite the pressures she observed in the ward areas, a result of shortened length of stay and reduced support services, when she asked nurses about the impact of these changes on their work, they could not provide concrete evidence of what nurses do and how restructuring was preventing them from doing it. Rather, nurses simply lamented a diminished ability to know patients as people and have relationships with them.

Weinberg argues that the nurses' accounts bore little resemblance to her observations of their work. Weinberg argues that while getting to know patients was an integral part of nurses' practice, this knowing did not involve friendliness or personal intimacy. Rather, '[k]nowing the patient involved learning about the physical and emotional dimensions of a patient's illness, finding out how the patient responded to treatment and managed complex medication regimens, and discerning what resources the patient would need to cope with their illness and treatment regimens one they left the hospital. Knowing the patient required familiarity with their medical record, with the care plans of other providers, with the patient's current physical and emotional state, and with the patient's home situation. Knowing the patient was a professional, not a personal activity' (p. 36). Weinberg concluded that while knowing the patient was central to nursing work, this was an instrumental relationship rather than one founded on emotional intimacy.

Weinberg argues that the nurses' focus on personal relationships prevented them from being able to explain how care was being threatened by the changes that were taking place in the organisation. Managers who were responsible for the restructuring were unaware of the real impacts of the organisational changes on nursing practice. Confronted with pictures of personal intimacy, managers concluded that time with patients was a luxury which the organisation could not afford and pressed ahead with their plans. The result? 'Although the nurses were becoming increasingly dissatisfied and suffering from burnout, they failed to articulate restructuring's negative effects and advocate for themselves and their patients. In a pattern increasingly prevalent in hospitals across the country, nurses were quietly choosing to leave the bedside and the profession rather than challenge financially motivated changes that endangered nurses and patients' (p. 31).

Gordon, S., 2006. The New Cartesianism: dividing mind and body and thus disembodying care. In: Nelson, S., Gordon, S. (Eds.), The Complexities of Care: Nursing Reconsidered. Cornell University Press, Ithaca and London, pp. 104–121.
Weinberg, D.B., 2006. When little things are big things: the importance of relationships for nurses' professional practice. In: Nelson, S., Gordon, S. (Eds.), The Complexities of Care: Nursing Reconsidered. Cornell University Press, Ithaca and London, pp. 30–43.

BOX 6.3 ■ Definition: Dirty Work

The concept of dirty work was introduced into the sociological literature by E.C. Hughes (1984). Hughes was interested in work, and in particular the commonalities of work across different occupations and professions. He understood an occupation to be comprised of a bundle of tasks. While not all the tasks in an occupation require the same level of skill or have the same value, they can be held together because they seem natural parts of a role or can most conveniently be performed together. Hughes argued that all occupations have a sense of their rightful tasks and functions. An activity within an occupational bundle can be valued above all others, but other tasks can be considered 'dirty' and threaten an individual's occupational identity.

Emerson and Pollner (1976) used ideas about dirty work in their research on community mental health professionals. They explored the designation of certain aspects of community mental health practice as 'shit work'. Whereas crisis intervention and avoiding hospitalisation were regarded as therapeutic work, involuntary detention was described as 'shit work' as it was primarily a mechanism of social control and served no therapeutic purpose.

Emerson, R.M., Pollner, M., 1976. Dirty work designations: their features and consequences in a psychiatric setting. Soc. Probl. 23(3), 243–254. doi:10.1525/sp.1976.23.3.03a00010.
Hughes, E.C., 1984. The Sociological Eye: Selected Papers. Transaction Books, New Brunswick and London.

---

and the relationship between failures of coordination and patient outcomes, it is self-evident that the work nurses do to hold together patient care constitutes a vital safety net in healthcare systems and represents a source of organisational resilience (see Chapter 5, Box 5.5). Not only does this reframing take seriously the organisational components of nursing practice, but it also invites critical consideration of the consequences of failing to formally acknowledge the importance of care trajectory management in the nursing role.

The Consequences of Invisibility

In the previous section, we considered the mechanisms through which work can be rendered visible or invisible, and how care trajectory management has been hidden from view by a professionalising strategy in which nursing's jurisdictional claims have centred on emotional intimacy and care-giving. In this section, we will consider the consequences of this invisibility and why it is important that care trajectory management is a fully integrated and formally recognised element of the nursing role.

NURSING WORK-AS-DONE IS NOT UNDERSTOOD

The first consequence of the invisibility of care trajectory management is that it impacts on societal understanding of nursing work. In 2009 the UK was rocked by evidence of a catastrophic breakdown in care standards in Mid Staffordshire NHS Trust. It was estimated that over a 5-year period, many patients died unnecessarily, and countless others experienced poor-quality care. In March 2009 a report from the Healthcare Commission, an independent inspector and regulator of health and social services in England, found that the standard of care at Mid Staffordshire was 'appalling'. This precipitated an independent public inquiry led by Robert Francis QC (Queen's Counsel). The Francis Reports (House of Commons, 2010, 2013) catalogue numerous examples of failings in care: patients' requests for assistance to use the bed pan or toilet going unheeded, people being left in soiled sheets for considerable periods of time, a high incidence of falls, neglected hygiene needs, failures in addressing patient requirements for nutrition and hydration, a disregard for privacy and dignity, poor communications and inadequate discharge management. But while Francis identified an extensive range of *system-wide* factors that contributed to these failings (Box 6.4), it was nurses that were pilloried in the press.

No professional cadre can have seen its public standing sink lower, and faster, than that of the nurse. The descendants of Florence Nightingale now lie somewhere between tabloid journalists and hedge funders in the public's estimation. Private Eye has started running a cartoon regular called 'fallen angels' in which the idiocies of modern nursing are parodied.

We hear seemingly endless stories of patients crying out in pain or thirst while being ignored, of the muddle-headed desire to professionalise what should always have been a vocational career, of nurses too proud to clean, to comfort, to sit and talk.

Hanlon (2012)

BOX 6.4 ■ Factors Identified as Contributing to the Failings at Mid Staffordshire NHS Trust in the Public Inquiry

The Trust Board did not listen to patients and staff to ensure the correction of deficiencies brought to the Trust's attention.

The Trust did not address a culture which tolerated poor standards and a disengagement from managerial and leadership responsibilities.

The Trust was focused on reaching national targets, achieving financial balance and seeking Foundation Trust status, at the cost of delivering acceptable standards of care.

The checks and balances which should have prevented such systemic failures also failed. The reasons for this include:

- The organisation was focused on doing the system's business—not that of the patients.
- An institutional culture which ascribed more weight to positive information about the service than to information capable of implying cause for concern.
- Standards and methods of measuring compliance which did not focus on the effect of a service on patients.
- A failure of communication between the many agencies to share their knowledge of concerns.
- Assumptions that monitoring, performance management or intervention was the responsibility of someone else.
- A failure to tackle challenges in building up a positive culture, in nursing in particular, but also within the medical profession.
- A failure to appreciate until recently the risk of disruptive loss of corporate memory and focus resulting from repeated, multilevel reorganisation.

NHS, National Health Service.

From House of Commons, 2013. Report of the Mid Staffordshire NHS Foundation Trust Public Inquiry, Volumes I, II and III (Chaired by Robert Francis QC), HC 898. The Stationery Office, London. https://www.gov.uk/government/publications/report-of-the-mid-staffordshire-nhs-foundation-trust-public-inquiry (Accessed 20 February 2023).

EXERCISE 6.1

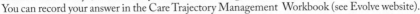

Imagine that you are stopped by a journalist to comment on the 'idiocies of modern nursing' as parodied in Private Eye, how would you describe nursing work?

You can record your answer in the Care Trajectory Management Workbook (see Evolve website).

What was so striking about the media onslaught triggered by the Mid Staffordshire scandal was that the leaders of nursing seemed quite unable to defend the profession or mount a convincing public response. Of course, it is very hard to defend poor nursing care, and nobody could fail to be shocked by the picture that emerged from the Francis Inquiry. But the issue is more complex than the task of defending the indefensible. One of the challenges that confronted the nursing leadership in the face of widespread criticism following the public inquiry was the growing gap between how the profession describes its practice and is perceived by the public and the reality of nursing work-as-done in contemporary healthcare systems (see, e.g., Traynor, 2014; Ajiboye, 2004; Staniszewska and Ahmed, 1998).

In the context of the Mid Staffordshire inquiry, the antiintellectualist arguments about preparation for nursing practice which were described in Chapter 1 resurfaced (see Box 1.3). The supposed deficiencies of graduate nurses were a consequence, it was claimed, of models of nurse education which focused on theory at the expense of practice and produced nurses lacking the skills and compassion of their predecessors trained in more traditional models (Hayter, 2013). In response to the Francis Report, and uncritically embracing such arguments, the UK government proposed that all prospective entrants to nursing should first work for a year as support workers or healthcare assistants as prerequisite for receiving funding for their degree. Although the changes were never implemented, when the Royal College of Nursing challenged the UK government's ill-informed response to the care scandal, it was quickly silenced by the accusation that it was not on the side of patients (Press Association, 2013).

In the wake of the Mid Staffordshire scandal, Ann Clwyd, a Labour Member of Parliament, was appointed by the then Prime Minister David Cameron to examine how the UK National Health Service (NHS) handled complaints. In an article reported in the UK national newspaper *The Independent*, it was claimed that she had received more than 2000 letters from patients, relatives and NHS staff and that one area of significant concern was nurses' stations (Wright, 2013).

People are incensed by nurses' stations. They say they just gather and chat constantly. They are suggesting bringing back the desk on the ward – not off the ward.

Clwyd suggested that removing nurses' stations completely and reintroducing desks in the middle of wards could have the effect of forcing nursing staff to interact more with patients and ensure higher standards of care. Of course, nurses' stations are places where teams gather and talk; they are the information hubs on hospital wards. It is where clinical records are reviewed and generated, information is retrieved and made sense of and phone calls are made to organise care. It is the space where referral forms are completed, and discharge summaries written. It is where second opinions are sought, and informal updates on patients' progress given. Not only is this legitimate work, it is important work, but it is clearly not widely recognised as such. It does not take place at the bedside; it is not direct patient care (Exercise 6.1).

THE CONTRIBUTION OF CARE TRAJECTORY MANAGEMENT TO HEALTHCARE QUALITY AND SAFETY IS NOT RECOGNISED

As the discussion of nurses' stations highlights, care trajectory management involves information seeking and information sharing and much of this work takes place away from the patient. Whether at the nurses' station in the acute setting, in a patient's home, in the car in between home visits or back at base in the community care team, this is essential work which requires time and cognitive capacity to be undertaken correctly. In *The Invisible Work of Nurses* (Allen, 2015), I observed that community nurses had decreasing opportunities for the documentation of care, with many undertaking this activity in their own time as their working days became filled with direct care work. In the acute sector, nurses were observed to stay beyond the end of their shift to complete care records. Ensuring adequate documentation is essential to communicate between members of the healthcare team; it is often the *only* information that is available to support transfers of care. It is safety critical work, but it is not treated as such. Consider the following example from *The Invisible Work of Nurses*:

Staff Nurse is looking through the unified assessment form for the purposes of finding information to include in the community nurse transfer letter. Most of the booklet is blank – only the face sheet data is entered. She flicks through the pages in a cursory manner. She is about to transfer the phone number when she notices that it has too many digits in it. She goes to the computer to cross-check and discovers that this is completely different, so she goes to speak to the patient. She returns, picks up the patient's notes and scrutinises the casualty card. She does not make any further entries into the transfer letter but sits leafing through the continuation sheets. She picks up her handover sheet from the desk and scrutinises this. She then enters information on the transfer letter in relation to past medical history which she has evidently been able to obtain from the handover sheet. She then moves on to scrutinise the discharge notification form and extracts further information which she includes in the transfer letter.

Whilst she is doing this, she answers the phone twice. On one occasion the call is from a social worker, and she passes the phone to her colleague who is sitting next to her also writing her notes. The second call is an inquiry after a patient being cared for by someone else. He is not at the Nurses' Station and Staff Nurse must leave the area to locate him. A few minutes later a medical consultant arrives on the ward and asks to see a patient. Staff Nurse directs him to the 9-bedded area. He asks for the patient's notes, and she points to the notes trolley.

(With permission from Taylor & Francis Group. Allen, D., 2015. The Invisible Work of Nurses: Hospitals, Organisation and Healthcare. Routledge, London and New York, pp. 122–123.)

When I was collecting data for *The Invisible Work of Nurses*, I was intrigued to observe that during medication rounds, nurses wore red tabards with 'do not disturb' printed on each face. This was a locally implemented safety initiative led by a clinical development practitioner who observed that when a nurse administered medications, they were interrupted up to 17 times. The intervention was intended to improve the safety of medicines administration and enable the nurse to concentrate without distraction. Over the last decade, several studies have reported interventions designed to reduce interruptions to nurses during the preparation and administration of medications (Bower et al., 2015; Flynn et al., 2016; Tomietto et al., 2012). These interventions are based on an underlying assumption that interruptions are significantly associated with medication administration errors. Accordingly, reducing interruptions should result in fewer medication administration errors and less harm to patients. There is little evidence to support the effectiveness of tabards in reducing interruptions on the medication round (Raban and Westbrook, 2014); however, the point to emphasise here is that the risks to patients associated with interruptions are recognised. Documentary work is not seen in the same way, but the consequences of getting this wrong are no less significant, even if the causal pathway is more complex. The growing volume of documentation in healthcare systems which does not add value further increases the danger that this essential safety critical work is trivialised or dismissed as just 'more paperwork' (Royal College of Nursing, 2013) (Exercise 6.2).

EXERCISE 6.2

List all the paper or digital documentation completed for the purposes of a patient admission in your clinical area. What functions does the paperwork serve? How is it used in the organisation of patient care during the patient's admission? Is anything missing? Is anything unnecessary? Which information is duplicated in different documents?

CARE TRAJECTORY MANAGEMENT IS NOT SUPPORTED BY HEALTHCARE INFORMATION AND COMMUNICATION INFRASTRUCTURES

Because of its invisibility, care trajectory management is not well served by existing healthcare information and communication infrastructures. Nurses often work within and around the systems imposed on them, rather than influencing their design and procurement, and regularly develop their own technologies to support their practice (Talamo et al., 2017).

Wisner et al. (2019) carried out an evidence synthesis on the impact of the electronic health record on nurses' cognitive work. Eighteen studies were included in the review which were analysed thematically. The authors found that most studies indicated the electronic record made it very difficult for nurses to develop an overview of the patient. It was challenging to assemble a chronology of events and to make sense of the implications of data. Information was fragmented and navigating the volume of material increased nurses' cognitive load. Summary reports and handoff tools in the electronic health record were insufficient to support nurses' work throughout the shift or for the purposes of handover, leading them to rely on self-made paper-based systems (Box 6.5). The authors note the importance of information management for the purposes of patient safety and argue that their findings have significant implications for the design of electronic health records.

Building on the findings of my review of field studies which highlighted the ubiquity of organising work in nursing practice (Chapter 1, Box 1.1), Talamo et al. (2017) used ethnographic methods to examine the patient and organisational aspects of the nursing role through the analysis of information and communication infrastructures. They found that the formal information technologies centred on the care of individual patients, whereas activities related to the organisational elements of nursing work were not supported by any official tools or systems in use. The gaps were addressed by nurses themselves in developing their own tools. The authors argue that the tools designed by the nurses supported the shifts in focus from the eye on the patient to the eye on the ward which, as described in Chapter 2, is part of nursing's distinctive nursing habitus (Bourdieu, 1980).

Nurses have often been reluctant to get involved in digital technologies (Booth et al., 2021), but through their care trajectory role, they have precisely the expertise that is necessary to inform the development of systems that support everyday work activity based on the work as it is done, rather than the work as it imagined. Digital engineers should be working with nurses to understand their own grown systems as the starting point for system development.

BOX 6.5 ■ Implementation of Electronic Handover

Ihlebæk (2020) studied the implementation of a computer-mediated handover—termed 'silent reporting'—in a Norwegian hospital cancer ward. The underlying idea of silent reporting is that all the information required for handover is made available in the electronic record, and thus, there is no requirement for ward nurses to meet face to face.

The research data were generated through 5 months of participant observation and nine semistructured interviews with nurses, who were selected to ensure representation by clinical experience. Observations revealed that further discussion was necessary to supplement the electronic handover related to the coordination of activity, including contextual information required for understanding the patient, which could not be captured in the formal record, resolution of uncertainty and ambiguities and joint decision making and problem solving. Ihlebæk argues that the study supports the findings of others that handover must be understood as more than patient information sharing, rather it is embedded in complex work practices, involving interactions with others.

Ihlebæk, H.M., 2020. Lost in translation – silent reporting and electronic patient records in nursing handovers: an ethnographic study. Int. J. Nurs. Stud. 109. doi:10.1016/j.ijnurstu.2020.103636.

CARE TRAJECTORY MANAGEMENT IS NOT COUNTED IN NURSING WORKLOAD MEASUREMENT SYSTEMS

The invisibility of care trajectory management has implications for decisions about workforce planning. There is growing international concern about nurse staffing levels and an accumulative body of evidence that points to the relationship between skill mix and the quality and safety of patient care (Aiken et al., 2013; Ball et al., 2014; Kane et al., 2007; Rafferty et al., 2007). A range of methods have emerged across the developed world for the purposes of determining optimal nurse staffing levels (establishment setting) and informing the daily deployment of staff in response to fluctuating demand patterns. These include professional judgement-based systems, simple volume-based systems (such as nurse-to-patient ratios), patient classification and time-task approaches (Griffiths et al., 2020). While there is limited evidence on which to select any specific method or tool (Griffiths et al., 2020), there is nevertheless an appetite for formal systems and tools to support practice and a growing acknowledgement of the merits of a triangulated approach, meaning that two or more recognised workforce planning methods to measure and model ward staffing should be used to increase the validity of the results (Royal College of Nursing, 2010).

While numerous tools exist for assessing nursing workload, these focus on direct patient care activity, typically expressed as a measure of patient acuity or care hours. Historically, the organisational component of nursing work has either been excluded from existing methodologies or, if acknowledged, it is either expressed as a 'professional judgement' about the wider contextual factors consequential for workload, or it is reflected in the use of proxy indicators, such as patient throughput, which lack the specificity of systematically generated numerical data. This means that, currently, nursing work is only partially recorded and therefore workload modelling and staff deployment fail to capture all aspects of the complexity and volume of nursing work. To offer some examples: Patients admitted for elective surgery would not be assessed as acutely ill or have high levels of dependency, but there is a significant volume of nursing activity associated with their preparation for surgery. Frail older patients awaiting discharge may have minimal nursing care needs, but high levels of work associated with organising their transition of care. Medical patients with uncertain diagnoses may require limited direct nursing care, but significant input associated with the organisation of tests and investigations and interactions with a range of medical specialists.

Capturing care trajectory management work is even more important in healthcare systems, such as the UK NHS, where extensive use is made of unqualified support staff. In staffing models of this kind, the assessment that the patient population has low levels of acuity without considering the work involved in managing their trajectories of care could result in an inappropriate support worker-registered nursing skill mix. It is not surprising that the organisational components of nursing work are regarded as a distraction from patient care if existing methodologies do not take this element of nursing work into account in calculating nurse staffing levels and skill mix.

UNCERTAIN LEGITIMACY AND AUTHORITY OF CARE TRAJECTORY MANAGEMENT WORK

Work is made visible through different indicators which change according to the context and perspective (Muller, 1999; Star and Strauss, 1999). Visible work tends to be equated with formal work that is authorised, and thus, the visibility of work is at the centre of politics about what will count as work (Hampson and Juror, 2005, 2010; Suchman, 1995). While *The Invisible Work of Nurses* (Allen, 2015) underlined the importance of nurses' care trajectory management for the quality and safety of patient care, it acknowledged that nurses often had uncertain authority in their work. The capacity of nurses to flourish in fulfilling their care trajectory management functions hinges to a considerable extent on the willingness of others to recognise the importance of this work. Some nurses worked in formal coordinator roles which conferred organisational legitimacy on their care trajectory management functions, but many others struggled to overcome organisational barriers

> **BOX 6.6 ■ The Uncertain Authority of Care Coordination in the Emergency Department**
>
> Wise et al. (2022) researched Emergency Department coordinators in Australia to better understand how they accomplished interprofessional coordination. The authors carried out 19 semistructured interviews with Emergency Department nurses, doctors and nurse practitioners, which were analysed thematically.
>
> A dominant institutional logic (see Chapter 3, Box 3.8) driving the organisation of Emergency Department work is ensuring the movement of patients through the system. This reflects the influence of performance targets, but also the requirement to ensure Emergency Department capacity to accept new patients. Emergency Department coordinators are charged with ensuring patient flow; they have an overview of department activity and are a central point of communication to ensure the mobilisation of patients' trajectories of care through the department.
>
> The research findings highlight the ambiguity of the coordinator role, which required coordinators to constantly renegotiate their authority to take the actions required to maintain the movement of patients through the Emergency Department. The authors conclude that better-defined nurse coordinator roles with clearer authority and clarity about 'who leads' interprofessional teams are required.
>
> Wise, S., Duffield, C., Fry, M., Roche, M., 2022. Nurses' role in accomplishing interprofessional coordination: lessons in 'almost managing' an emergency department team. J. Nurs. Manag. 30(1), 198–204.

and professional hierarchies to progress patient care. As research on nursing roles has identified, this uncertain authority needs to be addressed (Duffrey, 2017; Wise et al., 2022) (Box 6.6). If care trajectory management was a formally mandated nursing function, then healthcare organisations would confer upon others, including doctors, the obligation to align their own practices to such arrangements.

NURSES SUSTAIN FAULTY SYSTEMS RATHER THAN INTERVENING TO ADDRESS UNDERLYING ISSUES

A final consequence of the invisibility of nursing's care trajectory management function is that nurses often end up working around and propping up faulty systems rather than intervening to address the fundamental issues. Because frontline staff move quickly to compensate for system failures, underlying problems remain unacknowledged (Tucker, 2004) and dysfunctional systems and practices appear to be performing better than they are (Tucker, 2004; Tucker and Edmondson, 2003). This, as Wears and Hettinger (2013) put it, is the 'tragedy of adaptability'. Thus, while embracing the arguments from complexity science about the importance of frontline workers as sources of organisational resilience, it is important to maintain a critical awareness of the difference between unavoidable sources of unpredictability that stem from the work and avoidable sources of complexity which are the result of system dysfunction. Recognising the value of the organisational elements of nursing work necessitates looking beyond the management of care trajectories, to consider how the volume and complexity if this work can be reduced by improvements to the healthcare system.

Summary

This chapter has traced the history of nursing's professionalisation project and described how a strategy of expressing nursing's jurisdictional claims exclusively in terms of relationships with patients has rendered invisible large aspects of nursing practice, including nursing's care trajectory management function. This invisibility has tangible professional and practical consequences, for the everyday work of nurses and the wider contribution of the profession.

This chapter draws to a close Section I of this text. The last six chapters have ranged over a broad terrain to explore the professional and policy contexts which have shaped nursing practice over the last 50 years. The aim was to assemble an evidence-based case for formally integrating care trajectory management into the contemporary nursing jurisdiction (Allen, 2014). The first step in realising this aim is to expand nursing's professional vocabulary to enable practitioners, academics and nurse managers to better communicate the organisational elements of nursing work. The chapters that comprise Section II of this text are intended to furnish these theoretical and conceptual foundations and support their application to practice.

SUMMARY OF KEY LEARNING

- In progressing its status as a recognised profession, nursing's claim to jurisdiction has been expressed in terms of the nurse–patient relationship.
- While nursing's professionalisation strategy has been successful in unifying the work of a large and diverse profession, it has rendered invisible core nursing functions, including care trajectory management.
- The invisibility of care trajectory management has tangible consequences: nursing work is poorly understood by the public and policy makers, nursing work is inadequately supported in practice, and nurses often end up sustaining faulty systems, rather than intervening to improve them.
- Formal acknowledgement of nurses' care trajectory management function is essential for nursing to fully realise its contribution to the quality and safety of healthcare.

QUICK QUIZ

- In what way is care trajectory management functionally invisible work?
- What is professionalisation?
- What is jurisdiction?
- How have professionalisation processes in nursing rendered care trajectory management invisible?
- What is the tragedy of adaptability?

References

Abbott, A., 1988. The System of Professions: An Essay on the Division of Expert Labor. University of Chicago Press, Chicago, IL.

Aiken, L., Sloane, D.M., Bruyneel, L., Van den Heede, K., Sermeus, W.RN4CAST Consortium., 2013. Nurses' reports of working conditions and hospital quality of care in 12 countries in Europe. Int. J. Nurs. Stud. 50 (2), 143–153.

Ajiboye, P., 2004. What the public say. Nurs. Stand. 18 (17), 14–15.

Allen, D., 2001. The Changing Shape of Nursing Practice: The Role of Nurses in the Hospital Division of Labour. Routledge, London and New York.

Allen, D., 2004. Re-reading nursing and re-writing practice: towards an empirically based reformulation of the nursing mandate. Nurs. Inq. 11 (4), 271–283.

Allen, D., 2014. Reconceptualising holism within the contemporary nursing mandate: from individual to organisational relationships. Soc. Sci. Med. 119, 131–138.

Allen, D., 2015. The Invisible Work of Nurses: Hospitals, Organisation and Healthcare. Routledge, London and New York.

Armstrong, D., 1983. The fabrication of nurse-patient relationships. Soc. Sci. Med. 17 (8), 457–460.

Ball, J., Murrells, T., Rafferty, A.M., Morrow, E., Griffiths, P., 2014. 'Care left undone' during nursing shifts: associations with workload and perceived quality of care. BMJ Qual. Saf. 23 (2), 116–125. doi:10.1136/bmjqs-2012-001767.

Booth, G.R., Strudwick, G., McBride, S., O'Connor, S., López, S.A.L., 2021. How the nursing profession should adapt for a digital future. Br. Med. J. 373, n1190.

Bourdieu, P., 1980. The Logic of Practice. Stanford University Press, Stanford.

Bower, R., Jackson, C., Manning, J.C., 2015. Interruptions and medication administration in critical care. Nurs. Crit. Care. 20, 183–195. doi:10.1111/nicc.12185.

Buchan, J., Catton, H., Shaffer, F., 2022. The Global Nursing Workforce and the COVID-19 Pandemic. International Centre on Nurse Migration, Philadelphia, PA. https://www.icn.ch/system/files/2022-01/Sustain%20and%20Retain%20in%202022%20and%20Beyond-%20The%20global%20nursing%20workforce%20and%20the%20COVID-19%20pandemic.pdf (Accessed 1 December 2022).

Carpenter, M., 1977. The new managerialism and professionalism in nursing. In: Stacey, M., Reid, M., Heath, C., Dingwall, R. (Eds.), Health and the Division of Labour. Croom Helm, London, pp. 165–195.

Cavendish, C., 2013. The Cavendish Review: An Independent Review into Healthcare Assistants and Support Workers in the NHS and Social Care Settings. Department of Health and Social Care, England. https://assets.publishing.service.gov.uk/government/uploads/system/uploads/attachment_data/file/236212/Cavendish_Review.pdf (Accessed 20 January 2023).

Davies, C., 1995. Gender and the Professional Predicament in Nursing. Open University Press, Buckingham, UK.

Dingwall, R., Rafferty, A.M., Webster, C., 1988. An Introduction to the Social History of Nursing. Routledge, London.

Duffrey, P., 2017. Implementing the clinical nurse leader role in a large hospital network. Nurse Lead 15 (4), 267–280.

Flynn, F., Evanish, J.Q., Fernald, J.M., Hutchinson, D.E., Lefaiver, C., 2016. Progressive care nurses improving patient safety by limiting interruptions during medication administration. Crit. Care Nurse. 36, 19–35. doi:10.4037/ccn2016498.

Griffiths, P., Saville, C., Ball, J., Jones, J., Pattison, N., Monks, T., 2020. Safer Nursing Care Study Group, 2020. Nursing workload, nurse staffing methodologies and tools: a systematic scoping review and discussion. Int. J. Nurs. Stud. 103, 103487. doi:10.1016/j.ijnurstu.2019.103487.

Gordon, S., Nelson, S., 2006. Moving beyond the virtue script in nursing: creating a knowledge-based identity for nurses. In: Nelson, S., Gordon, S. (Eds.), The Complexities of Care: Nursing Reconsidered. Cornell University Press, Ithaca and London, pp. 13–29.

Hampson, I., Juror, A., 2005. Invisible work, invisible skills: interactive customer service as articulation work. New Technol. Work Employ. 20 (2), 166–181.

Hampson, I., Juror, A., 2010. Putting the process back in: rethinking service sector skill. Work Employ. Soc. 24 (3), 526–545.

Hanlon, M., 2012. First get rid of nurses' stations. https://hanlonblog.dailymail.co.uk/2012/12/first-get-rid-of-the-nursing-stations-.html (Accessed 12 December 2022).

Hart, E., 1991. A ward of my own: social organization and identity among hospital domestics. In: Holden, P., Littlewood, J. (Eds.), Anthropology and Nursing. Routledge, London, pp. 84–109.

Hayter, M., 2013. The UK Francis Report: the key messages for nursing. J. Adv. Nurs. 69 (8), e1–e3. doi:10.1111/jan.12206.

Hendrich, A., Chow, M., Skierczynski, B.A., Lu, Z., 2008. A 36-hospital time and motion study: how do medical-surgical nurses spend their time?. RCHE Publications 12 (3), 25–34.

Hendrickson, G., Doddato, T.M., Kovner, C.T., 1990. How do nurses use their time?. J. Nurs. Adm. 20 (3), 31–37.

Hollingsworth, J.C., Chisholm, C.D., Giles, B.K., Cordell, W.H., Nelson, D.R., 1998. How do physicians and nurses spend their time in the emergency department?. Ann. Intern. Med. 31 (1), 87–91.

House of Commons, 2010. Independent Inquiry Into Care Provided by Mid Staffordshire NHS Foundation Trust January 2005–March 2009, Volumes I and II (Chaired by Robert Francis QC), HC375. The Stationery Office, London. https://www.gov.uk/government/publications/report-of-the-mid-staffordshire-nhs-foundation-trust-public-inquiry (Accessed 20 February 2023).

House of Commons, 2013. Report of the Mid Staffordshire NHS Foundation Trust Public Inquiry, Volumes I, II and III (Chaired by Robert Francis QC), HC 898. The Stationery Office, London. https://www.gov.uk/government/publications/report-of-the-mid-staffordshire-nhs-foundation-trust-public-inquiry (Accessed 20 February 2023).

Hughes, E.C., 1984. The Sociological Eye: Selected Papers. Transaction Books, New Brunswick and London.

Kane, R.L., Shamliyan, T.A., Mueller, C., Duval, S., Wilt, T.J., 2007. The association of registered nurse staffing levels and patient outcomes: systematic review and meta-analysis. Med. Care. 45 (12), 1195–1204. doi:10.1097/MLR.0b013e3181468ca3.

Lawler, J., 1991. Behind the Screens: Nursing, Somology and the Problem of the Body. Churchill Livingstone, London.

May, C., 1992. Nursing work, nurses' knowledge, and the subjectification of the patient. Sociol. Health Illn. 14 (4), 472–487.

Muller, M.J., 1999. Invisible work of telephone operators: an ethnocritical analysis. Comput. Support. Coop. Work. 8, 31–61.

Nardi, B., Engeström, Y., 1999. A web on the wind: the structure of invisible work. Comput. Support. Coop. Work. 8, 1–8.

Nelson, S., Gordon, S., 2006. Introduction. In: Nelson, S., Gordon, S. (Eds.), The Complexities of Care: Nursing Reconsidered. Cornell University Press, Ithaca and London, pp. 1–12.

Perkin, H., 1989. The Rise of Professional Society: England Since 1880. Routledge, London.

Press Association, 2013. Cameron and Hunt hit back at RCN over nurse training reforms. https://www.the-guardian.com/society/2013/apr/22/cameron-hunt-rcn-nurse-training (Accessed 12 December 2022).

Raban, M.Z., Westbrook, J.I., 2014. Are interventions to reduce interruptions and errors during medication administration effective? A systematic review. BMJ Qual. Saf. 23, 414–421. doi:10.1136/bmjqs-2013-002118.

Rafferty, A.M., Clarke, S.P., Coles, J., Ball, J., James, P., McKee, M., et al., 2007. Outcomes of variation in hospital nurse staffing in English hospitals: cross sectional analysis of survey data and discharge records. Int. J. Nurs. Stud. 44, 175–182. doi:10.1016/j.ijnurstu.2006.08.003.

Royal College of Nursing, 2010. Guidance on Safe Nurse Staffing Levels in the UK. Royal College of Nursing, London.

Royal College of Nursing, 2013. Paperwork and Administration. Royal College of Nursing, London.

Staniszewska, S., Ahmed, L., 1998. Patient expectations and satisfaction with healthcare. Nurs. Stand. 12 (18), 34–38.

Star, S.L., Strauss, A., 1999. Layers of silence, arenas of voice: the ecology of visible and invisible work. Comput. Support. Coop. Work. 8, 9–30.

Suchman, L., 1995. Making work visible. Commun. ACM. 38 (9), 56–64.

Talamo, A., Mellini, B., Barbieri, B., 2017. The role of locally-designed organizational artifacts in supporting nurses' work: an ethnographic study on the wards. Prof. Inferm. 70 (2), 115–125.

Tomietto, M., Sartor, A., Mazzocoli, E., Palese, A., 2012. Paradoxical effects of a hospital-based, multi-intervention programme aimed at reducing medication round interruptions. J. Nurs. Manag. 20, 335–343. doi:10.1111/j.1365-2834.2012.01329.x.

Traynor, M., 2014. Caring after Francis: moral failure in nursing reconsidered. J. Res. Nurs. 19 (7–8), 546–556. doi:10.1177/1744987114557106.

Tucker, A.L., 2004. The impact of operational failures on hospital nurses and their patients. J. Oper. Manag. 22 (2), 151–169.

Tucker, A.L., Edmondson, A.C., 2003. Why hospitals don't learn from failures: organizational and psychological dynamics that inhibit system change. Calif. Manag. Rev. 45 (2), 55–72. doi:10.2307/41166165.

Wears, R.L., Hettinger, A.Z., 2013. The tragedy of adaptability. Ann. Emerg. Med. 63, 338–339.

Weinberg, D.B., 2006. When little things are big things: the importance of relationships for nurses' professional practice. In: Nelson, S., Gordon, S. (Eds.), The Complexities of Care: Nursing Reconsidered. Cornell University Press, Ithaca and London, pp. 30–43.

Westbrook, J.I., Duffield, C., Li, L., Creswick, N.J., 2011. How much time do nurses have for patients? A longitudinal study quantifying hospital nurses' patterns of task time distribution and interactions with health professionals. BMC Health Serv. Res. 11 (1), 1–12.

Wise, S., Duffield, C., Fry, M., Roche, M., 2022. Nurses' role in accomplishing interprofessional coordination: lessons in 'almost managing' an emergency department team. J. Nurs. Manag. 30 (1), 198–204.

Wisner, K., Lyndon, A., Chesla, C.A., 2019. The electronic health record's impact on nurses' cognitive work: an integrative review. Int. J. Nurs. Stud. 94, 74–84. doi:10.1016/j.ijnurstu.2019.03.003.

Wright, O., 2013. Get back on the ward: patients tsar tells nurses to talk less and care more. https://www.inde-pendent.co.uk/life-style/health-and-families/health-news/get-back-ward-patients-tsar-tells-nurses-talk-less-and-care-more-8555771.html (Accessed 12 December 2022).

Suggested Reading

The History of Nursing's Professional Development

Dingwall, R., Rafferty, A.M., Webster, C., 1988. An Introduction to the Social History of Nursing. Routledge, London.

Rafferty, A.M., 1996. The Politics of Nursing Knowledge. Routledge, London.

Both texts offer valuable insights into the politics of professionalisation processes in nursing history.

Care and Professional Identity

Nelson, S., Gordon, S. (Eds.), 2006. The Complexities of Care: Nursing Reconsidered. Cornell University Press, Ithaca and London.

An excellent collection of critical articles which challenge the assumption that nursing work is primarily emotional and relational.

Traynor, M., 2014. Caring after Francis: moral failure in nursing reconsidered. J. Res. Nurs. 19 (7–8), 546–556.

A discussion article, written in the aftermath of the Mid Staffordshire scandal, which considers the framing of failures of nursing care as moral failures.

Rethinking Nursing Jurisdiction

Allen, D., 2014. Re-conceptualising holism in the contemporary nursing mandate: from individual to organisational relationships. Soc. Sci. Med. 119, 131–138.

This paper summarises the main findings from *The Invisible Work of Nurses* Study to develop the case for reframing the contemporary nursing mandate to include the organisational as well as the clinical components of nursing practice.

SECTION II

The Theory and Practice of Care Trajectory Management

Section II introduces theories and concepts for the purposes of describing and explaining care trajectory management and illustrates their application to practice. It begins with the tenets and components of Translational Mobilisation Theory and outlines how these offer a framework for understanding the complexity of healthcare work and its organisation. These ways of seeing and understanding healthcare are then brought together into a framework which specifies and elucidates the practices of care trajectory management. The skills and knowledge underpinning care trajectory management are examined, and applied to a range of real-world scenarios.

CHAPTER 7

Conceptualising Healthcare Organisation for Care Trajectory Management

LEARNING OUTCOMES

At the end of this chapter, you will be able to:
- Outline the origins and development of translational mobilisation theory
- Explain the domain assumptions of translational mobilisation theory
- See the organisation of healthcare through the lens of translational mobilisation theory

Introduction

The next two chapters introduce Translational Mobilisation Theory (TMT) (Allen, 2018; Allen and May, 2017; https://www.translationalmobilisationtheory.org) and illustrate its application to healthcare. TMT has value for describing and understanding the complexity and organisation of healthcare work and provides the theoretical and conceptual foundations for the care trajectory management framework, which will be considered in Chapter 9. This chapter focuses on the underlying assumptions of TMT and shows how these offer a useful lens through which to comprehend and describe the everyday organisation of patient care. The core components of the theory will be explored in Chapter 8. Making an investment in understanding TMT and its application to healthcare is an important prerequisite for advancing care trajectory management in nursing practice. It offers a different way of seeing and describing the environments in which nurses practise (Allen, 2018) and lays the foundations for sharpening and perfecting nursing's professional vision (see Chapter 1, Making the Invisible, Visible: Why Concepts Matter for Nursing Practice).

The Development of Translational Mobilisation Theory

TMT is a sociological theory which explains the organisation of collective action in unpredictable work environments. TMT directs attention to how an activity is accomplished in everyday practice and the relationships between people, materials and technologies involved in achieving a shared goal (Box 7.1).

BOX 7.1 ■ Definition: Translational Mobilisation Theory

Translational Mobilisation Theory is a sociological theory of organisation which describes the relationships between people, materials and technologies in achieving a goal in dynamic systems of work.

Nowadays, few theories are developed from a blank slate. TMT draws on, reworks and synthesises elements of several sociological theories. These include the negotiated order perspective (Strauss et al., 1964), practice theories (Bourdieu, 1977; Engeström, 2000; Garfinkel, 1967; Giddens, 1984; Nicolini, 2012), ideas about actor networks (Latour, 2005), ecological approaches to the division of labour (Abbott, 1988; Freidson, 1976; Hughes, 1984; Strauss et al., 1985), Weick's (1969) insights on organisational sensemaking and the conceptualisation of strategic action fields laid out by Fligstein and McAdam (2011) (each of these theories is explained in more detail in Box 7.2).

BOX 7.2 ■ Theories Informing Translational Mobilisation Theory

Ecological Approaches to the Division of Labour

Ecological approaches to the division of labour have a long lineage in the sociology of work and occupations. They are founded on a shared understanding of the world of work as a dynamic system, comprised of occupations, technologies, workplaces, social problems and objects of practice, which interact with each other in response to changes in the wider environment. Ecological approaches have been deployed to consider the structure and function of the division of labour in society (Durkheim, 1933); the changing bundle of tasks through which occupations are established and their value in society (Abbott, 1988; Hughes, 1984); and how occupational roles, identities and jurisdictional boundaries are accomplished in the workplace (Allen, 1997, 2001; Freidson, 1976; Strauss et al., 1985).

The Negotiated Order Perspective

The negotiated order perspective is concerned with how meaning and order are created in organisations. It was developed by Strauss et al. (1963, p. 147–169) as a framework for conceptualising the ordered flux (Maines, 1982) they found in observational studies of two North American psychiatric hospitals between 1958 and 1962 (Strauss et al., 1964). Up to this point, theories of organisations had tended to emphasise the part of formal structures, processes and rules in ordering activity. Strauss et al. (1963) argued that organisational processes were more fluid than orthodox theories implied; people need to interact and negotiate with each other to accomplish their work and in so doing they both create and transform and are constrained by social structures (see also Chapter 4: Emergent Organisation).

Sensemaking in Organisations

Taking his point of departure from social psychology, Weick (1969) also advanced a process view of organisation, but whereas Strauss et al. (1964) underscored the importance of negotiation processes, Weick foregrounded organising. Weick (1969) was concerned with the cognitive and social processes through which organisational actors create order in conditions of complexity. This constellation of practices is encapsulated in the concept of *sensemaking*. Here, organisations take on a collective meaning in the interactions between the raw data of experience and the shared interpretative resources through which actors make sense of these experiences. This focuses attention on the interactions, communication and discourses as the sites in which organisation is enacted.

Practice Theory

Practice theory explains society in terms of activities and the things people do (Nicolini, 2012). It has its origins in a family of theories concerned with how human actions produce the social world, which includes praxeology (Bourdieu, 1977), ethnomethodology (Garfinkel, 1967), structuration (Giddens, 1984) and activity theory (Engeström, 2000). Practice theories understand social phenomena as constructed through action. Supposedly stable social structures—such as gender, a conversation or occupational role—are understood as verbs rather than nouns; they do not preexist human action, but are produced through it.

Practice theories emphasise that in making the social world real through everyday action, human subjects do not relate to the world directly; activities always involve artefacts. An artefact refers to an object, whether this is material or virtual, which is made by human beings. Practice approaches also draw attention to human

Continued

creativity, with practices understood as emerging from the interactions between people and the social and material world as individuals make sense of their circumstances and find creative solutions to problems.

Actor Network Theory

Actor network theory has its origins in sociological studies of science and technology but has been extended to a range of social phenomena (Latour, 2005). Actor network theory has two distinctive contributions to sociological theory. First, it understands social situations as shifting networks of assorted elements—people, technologies, devices, concepts, texts, materials, objects, statements. Second, both humans and nonhumans are regarded as having the capacity to 'act' within a network.

A central interest in actor network theory is with how social networks gain consistency and are maintained. Therefore, actor network theory informed research attends to the relationships in social situations and the mechanisms that hold the elements in a network together, either through the alignment of goals and concerns or by keeping contradictory components apart. *Translation* is the broad term used in actor network theory for these mechanisms.

Strategic Action Fields Theory

The concept of a strategic action field was developed by Fligstein and McAdam (2011) and is a synthesis of ideas drawn from scholarship in economic sociology, organisation studies and the sociology of social movements. Fligstein and McAdam argue that people are always acting strategically to create and maintain stable social worlds by securing the cooperation of others. The concept of a strategic action field refers to the conditions that shape collective action. Strategic action fields are constructed on a situational basis around a salient concern when actors (individual or collective) interact with knowledge of one another under a common set of understandings about the purposes of the field, the relationships in the field (including who has power and why) and the field's rules (Fligstein and McAdam, 2011, p. 3). Strategic action fields always operate in a larger political, economic and social context; like a Russian doll, open one up and it contains other strategic action fields.

Abbott, A., 1988. The System of Professions: An Essay on the Division of Expert Labor. University of Chicago Press, Chicago, IL.

Allen, D., 1997. The nursing-medical boundary: a negotiated order? Sociol. Health Illn. 19(4), 498–520.

Allen, D., 2001. The Changing Shape of Nursing Practice: The Role of Nurses in the Hospital Division of Labour. Routledge, London and New York.

Bourdieu P., 1977. Outline of a Theory of Practice. Cambridge University Press, Cambridge, UK.

Durkheim, E., 1933. The Division of Labour in Society. Collier-Macmillan Ltd, London.

Engeström, Y., 2000. Activity theory as a framework for analysing and redesigning work. Ergon. 43, 960–972.

Fligstein, N., McAdam, D., 2011. Toward a general theory of strategic action fields. Sociol. Theory. 29, 1–26.

Freidson, E., 1976. The division of labour as social interaction. Soc. Probl. 23, 304–313.

Garfinkel H., 1967. Studies in Ethnomethodology. Prentice Hall, Englewood Cliffs, NJ.

Giddens A., 1984. The Constitution of Society: Outline of a Theory of Structuration. Polity Press, Cambridge, UK.

Hughes, E.C., 1984. The Sociological Eye: Selected Papers. Transaction Books, New Brunswick, NJ, and London.

Latour, B., 2005. Reassembling the Social: An Introduction to Actor-Network-Theory. Oxford University Press, Oxford.

Maines, D., 1982. In search of mesostructures: studies in the negotiated order. Urban Life. 11, 278–279.

Nicolini, D., 2012. Practice Theory, Work, and Organization: An Introduction. Oxford University Press, Oxford.

Strauss, A., Fagerhaugh, S., Suczet, B., Wiener, C., 1985. Social Organization of Medical Work. University of Chicago Press, Chicago, IL.

Strauss, A., Schatzman, I., Bucher, R., Ehrlich, D., Sabshin, M., 1963. The hospital and its negotiated order. In: Freidson, E. (Ed.), The Hospital in Modern Society. Free Press, New York.

Strauss, A.L., Schatzman, L., Bucher, R., Ehrlich, D., Sabshin, M., 1964. Psychiatric Ideologies and Institutions. The Free Press of Glencoe Collier-Macmillan, London.

Weick, K.E., 1969. The Social Psychology of Organizing. Random House, London.

BOX 7.3 ■ Example of a Grounded Theory in Healthcare: Awareness Context Theory

Awareness context theory refers to the different levels of awareness of participants in an interaction about the health status of a patient, along with what the patient knows about others' awareness of their condition. It was developed by Glaser and Strauss (1965) based on comprehensive qualitative sociological research on the process of dying in six San Francisco Bay area hospitals in the 1960s. In *closed awareness contexts*, the patient does not know the status of their condition, whereas healthcare staff are fully informed. In *open awareness contexts*, everyone is aware of the condition of the patient. Although open awareness contexts are more typical in contemporary healthcare systems, this was not the case when the study was undertaken. Indeed, Glaser and Strauss were struck by how little patients knew about their impeding death. By drawing attention to the different awareness context that exists in the dying process, the research supported activists in improving the rights of dying patients (Timmermans, 2007). While there have been profound changes to the norms and expectations regarding information sharing in healthcare in the intervening period, these ideas have continued to have value in healthcare research and practice. For example, Timmerman (1994) further developed the theory to accommodate how patients and relatives emotionally cope with terminal information; Hellström et al. (2005) extended the concept to examine the impact of dementia on the everyday life and relationships of older spousal couples; and Stacey et al. (2019) deployed the concept to critically examine how the increased specialisation of healthcare and the fragmentation of services undermine the open awareness contexts considered to be the gold standard in contemporary healthcare systems.

Glaser, B.G., Strauss, A.L., 1965. Awareness of Dying. Aldine Transaction, New Brunswick, NJ.
Hellström, I., Nolan, M., Lundt, U., 2005. Awareness context theory and the dynamics of dementia: improving understanding using emergent fit. Dementia. 4, 269–295.
Stacey, C.L., Pai, M., Novisky, M.A., Radwany, S.M., 2019. Revisiting 'awareness contexts' in the 21st century hospital: how fragmented and specialized care shape patients' awareness of dying. Soc. Sci. Med. 220, 212–218.
Timmermans, S., 1994. Dying of awareness: the theory of awareness contexts revisited. Sociol. Health Illn. 16(3), 322–339. doi:10.1111/1467-9566.ep11348751.
Timmermans, S., 2007. Awareness Contexts. The Blackwell Encyclopaedia of Sociology. John Wiley & Sons, Ltd., Hoboken, NJ. doi:10.1002/9781405165518.

TMT is a grounded theory (Glaser and Strauss, 1967). This term is used to refer to theories that are developed from, and grounded in, empirical evidence, rather than arising from abstraction, or what is colloquially referred to as 'armchair theorising'. TMT was developed from *The Invisible Work of Nurses* study (Allen, 2015) and builds on a cumulative body of research on healthcare organisation (Allen, 2001, 2009; Allen et al., 2004a, 2004b), some of which is referred to for illustrative purposes in this text. Like most grounded theories, TMT is also a theory of the middle range. Middle range theories typically address a practical issue and have a more restricted focus than 'grand' theories of abstract phenomenon, such as 'power', 'gender' or 'social class'. Awareness context theory (Glaser and Strauss, 1965) is a classic example of a middle range grounded theory in healthcare (Box 7.3). More recent examples include normalisation process theory (May and Finch, 2009), a theory of how interventions become embedded in everyday practices derived from a programme of research on the implementation of healthcare technologies, and burden of treatment theory (May et al., 2014), which you were introduced to in Chapter 3 (see Box 3.2), and which focuses on the work required of patients and families as part of their ongoing healthcare management, and the implications this has for adherence to treatment regimes.

The Domain Assumptions of Translational Mobilisation Theory

Every theory is based on a perspective, a way of seeing and not seeing the world; this is typically referred to as a theory's *domain assumptions*. TMT is based on four domain assumptions which is important to understand in applying the theory. These overarching background beliefs set the foundations for understanding how healthcare is organised for the purposes of care trajectory management.

DOMAIN ASSUMPTION 1: AN ECOLOGICAL APPROACH TO THE ORGANISATION OF COLLECTIVE ACTION

TMT takes an ecological approach to the organisation of collective action (see Box 7.2). It focuses on the relationships between people, materials and technologies involved in a shared activity and how these interact and are shaped by the local context, or what Fligstein and McAdam (2011) call the strategic action field. For the purposes of care trajectory management, this domain assumption encourages an understanding of healthcare organisation as a complex dynamic system rather than a machine, where the whole is more than the sum of its parts and where the interaction between actors can produce unpredictable outcomes.

I was a member of a team which used an ecological approach to analyse the interactions between health and social care providers, patients and families, in research on interprofessional working in people who had suffered an acute stroke (Allen et al., 2004a, 2004b). Healthcare policy emphasises the centrality of individually tailored packages of care negotiated in partnership with users and carers and, where appropriate, characterised by interagency collaboration and team working. By adopting an ecological lens, we highlighted how care trajectories can be shaped by the social positioning and priorities of participants. In case of Edward Murphy, for example, interprofessional and intraprofessional disagreements, disagreements between members of the multidisciplinary team and families, and disagreements between different members of the same family were critical in conditioning the negotiation of Edward's discharge arrangements (Case Study 7.1).

CASE STUDY 7.1 Edward Murphy

Edward Murphy was admitted to hospital with sudden loss of speech, then loss of coordination. He had suffered a left frontal lobe infarction resulting in a right hemiplegia (paralysis) and dysphasia (difficulties in processing and formulating language). Edward was in his early forties and married, with one son. Edward's wife, Rhondda, was pregnant with twins. On admission Edward was completely dependent on nursing staff. He was immobile, incontinent and unable to comprehend any auditory or visual information. Two weeks later he began to develop some awareness and started to mobilise with the physiotherapists. However, although his dysphasia had improved, Edward had profound communication difficulties. Over the course of his inpatient care, both Edward and his wife suffered from depression and the multidisciplinary team often disagreed as they struggled to negotiate satisfactory arrangements for Edward and his family. During Edward's 8 months in the hospital, a variety of care arrangements was explored, ranging from discharge to home through to placement with a foster family. He was eventually placed in a residential home, where he settled well, attending the day hospital for therapy once a week.

The participants involved in Edward's case were Edward; Rhondda (Edward's wife); Edward's son, parents, sister and sister-in-law; consultant; speech and language therapist (SALT); senior occupational therapist; occupational therapist; social worker; relief social worker (R.SW); two senior house officers; senior physiotherapist; physiotherapist; chiropodist; two residential home proprietors; day centre nursing staff; day centre doctor; dermatologist; senior staff nurse; deputy ward manager; and a 'PP Homes' manager. They were representatives from a complex field which encompassed an acute NHS Trust, local authority social services organisation and the private care home sector. This meant that negotiations about Edward's discharge arrangements crossed interagency boundaries with different cultures, finances, geographical scope, management structures, priorities, professional allegiances and planning cycles and were conditioned by the limited support and facilities for young disabled people.

The team involved in Edward's case disagreed about the goals for discharge. On one side were Edward and the SALT who wanted a home discharge. On the other, his wife and the social worker claimed that with a young family to care for, Rhondda would be unable to cope with Edward at home and the discharge would be unsafe.

These issues were discussed at a case conference called by the SALT, which included all members of the multidisciplinary team, Rhondda (RM) and Edward's son and sister-in-law. The meeting began with the SALT explaining to the family that the purpose of the case conference was to 'decide with the family and everybody where Edward is going to go' following discharge. The SALT acknowledged Rhondda's concerns and argued that it was important to reach a decision about Edward's discharge destination so that time and effort were not wasted on planning, if returning home was not a viable option. However, despite her even-handed presentation of the meeting's purpose, throughout the discussion, the SALT was at pains to express her preferred position or goal (a home discharge) and/or undermine Rhondda's justification for her decision not to have Edward home. This is illustrated in the following extract, in which the conversation focused on Edward's communication problems:

SALT to RM: It's the communication that bothers you most.
RM: Mmm. Yeah, because it's no, you can't have a [...] he can't come up and tell me. You know? 'I want this' or you know? [...] He couldn't tell me 'I'm tired' or 'I've got a pain here'. He can't describe things to me.
SALT: What about then if you asked him questions based on what you think it might be?
RM: Yeah, but I'm there forever aren't I ((Gives an example)) [...]
SALT: So, you couldn't live with that level of pressure?
RM: (.) See, I don't know. I don't know, like I can't say what he would be like at home?
(Case Conference—audio recording)

Here then, the SALT positions Rhondda with responsibility for the problems of agreeing a discharge: it is her inability to cope with the pressure of managing Edward's communication difficulties that has placed the discharge arrangements in jeopardy.

The discussion then focuses on community support, which the R.SW explains is rather limited: a day centre is available some days a week but no home care. The scenario described by the social worker indicates a starker view of the reality of taking Edward home than that portrayed by the SALT, and this prompts the SALT to relinquish her preferred option. In so doing, however, it is Rhondda's inability to cope rather than the lack of support available to her that she presents as the decisive factor:

R.SW: But erm (.) I think you've got to be aware that if we are going with the home situation, the responsibility is going to be levelled on your shoulders for most of the time. [...] So you've got to know what you're taking on and, you know, what the situation is. [...] It is a permanent responsibility to know where we're going with that. And I think it is necessary for us to work with that because, you know, for something to last, or be OK for a couple of months, isn't any good. Because we're not talking about a couple of months.
SALT: Well, if that is the case, Rhondda, basically you're saying that you can't have him home. I'm not trying to put words in your mouth, but we have to be clear about what the options are.
(Case conference—tape recording)

The meeting is then refocused to consider what new arrangements are required to make progress in Edward's case. Despite the apparent agreement reached at the case conference meeting that Edward would be unable to return home, throughout the duration of his hospital admission, key members of the multidisciplinary team continued to press for this outcome. The following discussion takes place 2 months after the case conference:

SALT: I suggested to Raquel (relief social worker) that since his communication has improved a little, perhaps she would reconsider whether she (Rhondda) would have him at home. [...]
Senior staff nurse: I've spoken to her, and she said no way.
SALT: And what's her reason this time?
Senior staff nurse: Still that she's got a lot on her plate. That she's now nearly, nearly due [...] and he's not going to have time to settle in.
(Multidisciplinary team meeting—field notes)

The tension between the SALT and Rhondda is very evident in these data. Notice, in the previous extract, how the SALT subtly undermines Rhondda's credibility through the implication that her 'reasons' not to have Edward home are situated and shifting, i.e., excuses, rather than being founded on substantive concerns. Edward's case was also shaped by the existence of a strained relationship between his wife and his own relatives: Rhondda's decision not to have Edward home was informed by the belief that she would receive no help from Edward's family:

RM: Well, like I say (.) well because as you say, [...] the care is not going to be there, it will be me (.) then, you know? Obviously, his family is not here ((attending case conference)), which is a prime example. So, erm, you know?
(Case conference—audio recording)

Continued

The disagreements over Edward's discharge arrangements resulted in the development of conflictual elements between participants in his trajectory of care. For example, certain members of the multidisciplinary team expressed suspicion that Rhondda was attempting to use Edward's condition to assist her application for rehousing even though a decision appeared to have been taken that he was not going home:

Senior occupational therapist: His wife rang our main department this week. She wanted to have a copy of my home visit report, regarding housing (.) And she's seen me since but hasn't acknowledged this, so it's all a bit peculiar. Whether she's trying to go ahead with the housing situation regardless of where he's going. I'm not sure. [...]
Senior staff nurse: I think she is still using his case as the reason to get re-housed.
(Multidisciplinary team meeting—audio recording)

As researchers we were unable to establish the veracity of these claims; nevertheless, it is possible to see in this extract an example of the way in which an account of Edward's wife's motives is constructed which clearly questions any notion of her having Edward's best interests at heart. Rhondda's behaviour is formulated as both dishonest and governed by self-interest, as she uses 'his case as the reason to get rehoused'. Thus, a kind of moral blaming is taking place whereby her refusal to support the favoured outcome and care for her husband at home is linked to other proffered information, which is selectively interpreted, to question her character. This representation of Rhondda's motives discredits her as a participant in the planning process and can justifiably be disregarded by those who remain committed to the goal of determining the 'best' outcome for Edward.

The disagreements in Edward's case led to divisions and the formation of alliances within the team. Central to this was Edward's relationship with the SALT. Owing to his communication difficulties, the SALT took a lead role in his case and was a strong advocate for Edward throughout. In addition, when Rhondda indicated her reluctance to have Edward home, the SALT and other team members attempted to establish an alliance with Edward's parents to achieve their preferred objectives:

Senior occupational therapist: We wanted to get his parents involved. His wife was talking about sending him to London. His parents live in South Wales, and I don't think they'd be happy with that. So, we want to give them the option. We don't want them to turn around at a later date and say 'Nobody asked us what we wanted'. It'll be good to get them involved anyhow because it'd be awful for him to feel abandoned.
(Field notes)

In the event, the attempt to secure a co-operative relationship with Edward's parents was unsuccessful. The family arrived late for the crucial case conference, by which time all the key decisions had been made. Realising that her decision had alienated her from certain members of the multidisciplinary team, Rhondda formed an alliance with the social worker, who was more sympathetic to her situation.
Relief social worker: Rhondda is aware that she's become the villain of the piece.
SALT: What, on the unit?

Relief social worker: Yes. She's not stupid. She's confided in me about having him back. It would be the easiest thing in the world for her to have him back, to go along with everything and pretend there's no problem. But she's being very wise.
(Field notes)

Notice the contrast between this version of Rhondda's behaviour—'she's being very wise'—and that produced by the hospital-based team in the previous extract—'she's using him to get rehoused'. The social worker's alliance with Rhondda continued to be a powerful influence on Edward's trajectory and served to bring the direction of Edward's care plan closer to what was desirable to Rhondda despite what was by now a clear challenge from the SALT (supported by some members of the hospital team) as to what might be the best outcome in this case.

The disagreements within the multidisciplinary team, and between certain team members and Edward's wife, resulted in a struggle to control the pace of the decision-making processes about Edward's discharge arrangements. This was evident during the case conference meeting. Ordinarily, it is the social worker who would take the lead role in organising discharge; however, as Edward's self-appointed advocate, the SALT adopted an assertive role by seizing the initiative when it became apparent that Rhondda did not wish to have Edward home:

SALT: So, erm, my next issue really is because of his communication (.) we need to get across to Edward that this is the situation before we think about offering him other situations and see what there is. He's to be given the opportunity to say what he feels about that.
RM: Yeah.
SALT: [...] I think that that is probably the next move. [...] But because of his understanding problem we still have to take time to get that across to him rather than whisk him away and put him somewhere where he's not really come to terms with the fact that he's not going home.

(Case conference—audio recording)

It is at this point that it emerged that the R.SW and Rhondda have already arranged to visit alternative accommodation and, despite the SALT's efforts to control the pace of the process, the R.SW offers a different plan, retaining control over the timing of events:

R.SW: Well, I've already spoken to Rhondda about Cheshire Homes which (.) I've made quite a lot of enquiries and to my mind it's the only option for him. [...] It's thin on the ground that cater for people in residential setting with disabilities...[...] Rhondda has already made arrangements to go this afternoon...
SALT: Oh, right.
R.SW: ....to have a look at it. So, we let you go ahead with that. Encourage you to go ahead and ask all the questions you want. And then come back to me and say what your impressions are, because, correct me if I'm wrong, say for instance that you hated it and you thought, 'No, this is not the place for Edward.' You know? We'd have to rethink things completely. So, at this stage, I don't think it would be, erm, (.) constructive to start the process of Edward understanding about the home situation.'

(Case conference—audio recording)

It then emerged that the SALT was about to go on holiday for 2 weeks. It is possible therefore that her position was informed by her desire to ensure that Edward was informed of his wife's decision before starting annual leave. After some discussion, however, it was agreed that nothing more would be communicated to Edward until Rhondda had visited alternative accommodation and the SALT had returned from her holiday.

Despite the agreement reached at the case conference not to communicate anything to Edward until there was more certainty over the arrangements, the SALT went ahead and informed Edward about his wife's decision not to have him home. She also failed to inform Rhondda or other key members of the multidisciplinary team in the case of her actions:

Senior staff nurse: Megan (SALT, who is now on holiday) told him (about his wife's decision not to have him home). But unfortunately, nobody had phoned his wife to tell her that he knew they were no longer going to be together. And of course, then she came in on Tuesday not knowing what was wrong with him and he was all upset. [...] She went ballistic, that it was unprofessional, that he shouldn't have been told, if he was told, somebody should have called her and told her. And she's not happy with the whole situation at all.

(Multidisciplinary team meeting—audio recording)

It emerged that the R.SW was also unaware of the SALT's actions. The following extract reports on a conversation between the social worker and occupational therapists about Edward's case:

R.SW: Since from the meeting we'll have a fortnight while Megan (SALT) is away because nothing....everything is in limbo until Megan comes back because nobody is even remotely thinking. Even if she'd gone there and thought it was wonderful, nobody was gonna tell him anything about it until Megan is back.
Senior occupational therapist: (Peggy, who has overheard our conversation, interjects): He has been told.
R.SW: He has?!
Senior occupational therapist: Yeah, he has because Megan couldn't go away without telling him. He knew something was up. So she has told him that Rhondda cannot have him at home.
R.SW: Right.
Senior occupational therapist: There was no way that she could leave it because she came out of the meeting and he knew something was going on.
R.SW: Right. And so she's told him. Right, in that case ...
Senior occupational therapist: If you want to look in his medical notes, she's written a whole thing on it.
R.SW: Is he all right?
Senior occupational therapist: He's been OK.

Continued

CASE STUDY 7.1   Edward Murphy—cont'd

Occupational therapist: He's indicated his own wishes as well, in terms of where he wants to go. She's written it all down. [...]
R.SW: Right. Well I'm glad you told me that. I was not aware of that. Erm, Rhondda wasn't either was she because (.) she was under the impression that he didn't know anything about this at the moment. So she needs to be told that because obviously it's going to present an awkwardness between them. He knows what she's thinking, but she doesn't know that he knows that she knows.
Senior occupational therapist: Well, if you're happy to tell her that's fine. [...]
Occupational therapist: I think that what it was, when they finished the meeting Rhondda walked straight past him. And he could see that she was in floods of tears. And obviously she didn't make any attempt to speak with him, so
R.SW: Right. Right. So matters sort of came to a head. Well, anyway, that's life isn't it.

(Fieldnotes—audio-recorded conversation)

Rhondda and the multidisciplinary team explored several options for Edward when it was decided that he would not be returning home. They finally settled on the 'PP Home', a specialist facility designed to encourage independent living. As Edward's discharge date approached, however, it emerged that the 'PP Home' would be unavailable as there had been a delay in vacating the place he had been allocated. Edward was aggrieved by this turn of events and alternative arrangements in a residential care home had to be organised temporarily. Within a week of his discharge, a 'PP Home' place then became available. Having settled into alternative accommodation and dissatisfied by the withdrawal of the original offer, Edward refused the place. His communication difficulties meant that he had been excluded from participating in many of the meetings to discuss his future but in this case the decision to remain was his own. At the end of the study, Edward had settled well into his new accommodation from where he attended the day hospital for therapy once a week.

(With permission from Allen, D., Griffiths, L., Lyne, P., 2004a. Understanding complex trajectories in health and social care provision. Sociol. Health Ill., 26 (7): 1008–1030.)

Edward's discharge process might have been simpler and less protracted had the divisions between the participants not existed, but this would not necessarily have produced the best outcome for him and his family. Had the SALT's view prevailed, then Edward might have been discharged home without due consideration of the sustainability of these arrangements and the consequences for his wife and children. Although these questions are unanswerable, it is important to reflect upon them. For our immediate purposes, however, Edward's case highlights how the dynamics between participants operating within the constraints of the environment impact on the evolution of patient care trajectories in ways which cannot always be predicted. This ecological understanding of collective action is the first domain assumption of TMT.

DOMAIN ASSUMPTION 2: A PROCESS VIEW OF ORGANISATION

TMT is founded on a process view of organisation, informed by the negotiated order perspective (Strauss et al., 1963) and insights on organisational sensemaking (Weick, 1969) (see Box 7.2). From this perspective, supposedly stable organisational structures—such as professional roles, hierarchies or service processes—only come to life through the negotiations and sensemaking actions of organisational actors. In healthcare, the formal components of organisation are typically treated as external drivers of activity, but TMT conceptualises this relationship differently. Within the framework, human action and the formal features of healthcare organisation are treated as moving backwards and forwards in a dynamic relationship in 'a world that is always on the move' (Hernes, 2014). While formal structures are understood to shape the possibilities for action, their meanings are enacted by human agents through their use in practice. This domain assumption invites us to recognise the agency of participants in organisations and to understand the normal condition of healthcare organisation as an ongoing dynamic tension between stability and fluidity, and formality and informality, as the people who work in the system *negotiate* and *make sense of* the resources, opportunities and constraints, in carrying out their activities in response to the demands of a situation (Box 7.4; see Chapter 4, Box 4.2).

BOX 7.4 ■ The Changing Shape of Nursing Practice

In the 1990s, two major policy initiatives were introduced into the UK which had significant implications for the scope of nursing practice. First, the requirement to reduce the hours worked by junior doctors as part of the European Working Time Directive provided the impetus for extension of the nursing role to enable nurses to undertake tasks—such as venepuncture and intravenous infusions—which had previously been restricted to doctors. Second, the Project 2000 reforms of nurse education reduced learners' contribution to service provision from 60% to 20% and led to an increase in healthcare support workers. In responding to these seismic shifts in the policy landscape for nursing practice, the UK nursing regulator (United Kingdom Central Council) produced 'The Scope of Professional Practice' (UKCC, 1992). This guidance ended the requirement for nurses to secure medically sanctioned certificates to undertake tasks not covered in initial nursing training and shifted the responsibility for managing the boundaries of their practice onto individual nurses. In effect, nurses were directed to extend the scope of their practice to include medically delegated activities only if they were competent to perform the tasks in question and in doing so this did not result in the inappropriate shifting of nursing care activities, for which qualified staff were still formally responsible, to support workers.

I studied these processes as they were implemented in a surgical and a medical ward in a UK district hospital. I was interested in understanding how nurses accomplished their scope of practice *in practice*, and the situational considerations that impacted these decisions. My aim was to document occasions when nurses negotiated their role boundaries with medicine and support staff, to analyse how these were conditioned by context and the issues at stake. When I started the fieldwork, there was, however, very little to see, or at least at the level of everyday practice. In fact, the study revealed that the implementation of these policies largely formalised preexisting informal blurring of professional boundaries at both the nursing–medical and nursing–support worker interfaces which had been driven by the practical requirements of progressing patient care. Beyond the frontline, however, at the level of hospital management, implementing these changes generated a range of 'boundary work' strategies which reaffirmed the distinctive contributions and power relationships of medicine, nursing and support staff, in formal organisational structures, policies and procedures, despite the material changes in activity in the workplace.

From Allen, D., 1997. The nursing-medical boundary: a negotiated order? Sociol. Health Illn. 19(4), 498–520; Allen, D., 2001. The Changing Shape of Nursing Practice: The Role of Nurses in the Hospital Division of Labour. Routledge, London and New York.
UKCC, 1992. The Scope of Professional Practice. UKCC, London.

EXERCISE 7.1

Identify any areas of role overlap with other healthcare workers (doctors, administrative staff, healthcare support workers, catering staff, cleaners, porters). How do you negotiate these role boundaries in everyday practice?
You can record your answer in the Care Trajectory Management Workbook (see Evolve website).

This relationship between formal structures and everyday negotiations is captured in the aphorism 'health services work despite the system'. The effects of these ways of working can be both positive and negative of course. Research on the implementation of innovations in healthcare highlights how interventions become embedded in organisations because of the negotiations, workarounds and tinkering work that people do to integrate them into practice for patient benefit (Timmermans and Berg, 2003), and insights from coroners' Prevention of Future Deaths reports highlight inappropriate adherence to protocols as a system error (Leary et al., 2021). On the other hand, however, such practices can lead to normalised deviance and have a negative impact on healthcare quality (Banja, 2010; Barach and Phelps, 2013) (Exercise 7.1).

DOMAIN ASSUMPTION 3: ACTIVITY IS MEDIATED BY ARTEFACTS

The third domain assumption of TMT, derived from practice theory (see Box 7.2), is that human activity is always mediated by artefacts. Artefacts can be material—such as tools or machines—or

---

BOX 7.5 ■ Plugging Information Technology Gaps for Care Trajectory Management

In one ward in *The Invisible Work of Nurses* (Allen, 2015) study, there was an A4 hardbacked book which functioned as a real-time summary of each patient's care. It was easily transportable and could be quickly updated during ward rounds and interactions with other members of the healthcare team, with different coloured ink used to revise the record so that changes were readily identifiable. The ward book enabled an overview of each patient's care which was not available anywhere else in the information and communications infrastructure, but which was essential in supporting trajectory management. While reflecting the logic of nurses' organising work, technologies such as this operated under the radar of formal organisational processes and, lacking legitimacy, were not integrated into management and information systems.

Allen, D., 2015. The Invisible Work of Nurses: Hospitals, Organisation and Healthcare. Routledge, London and New York.

---

they can be cognitive—such as categories, concepts or rules of thumb. They can be formal or informal. Focusing on formal artefacts draws attention to objects that are mandated by an organisation. Focusing on informal artefacts focuses attention to the creativity of participants in developing objects to support their practice. The latter tend to be based on the needs of the work-as-done and highlight gaps in formal provision (see Chapter 6, Care Trajectory Management Is Not Supported by Healthcare Information and Communication Infrastructures).

As you learnt in Chapter 3 (see, Complexity 2: Healthcare Is Technologically Rich), healthcare work involves a wide array of material artefacts. Examples include highly sophisticated technologies such as scanners, through everyday technologies such as whiteboards, monitoring equipment and computers, extending to mundane technologies, such as pens and paper. In addition to the formal technologies that support healthcare work, participants may use informal material artefacts to support practice, such as the 'scraps' deployed by nurses to manage patient care work reported by Hardey et al. (2000), the ward books I observed in the *Invisible Work of Nurses* (Allen, 2015) (Box 7.5) or the medication organisers or blood sample planners described by Talamo et al. (2017).

Healthcare is also awash with formal cognitive artefacts, that is, artefacts developed to support mental processes. A cursory glance through a patient's medical record will likely reveal a very wide range—risk assessment scores (falls, manual handling, pressure injury), triage assessments, laboratory results, patient experience data, early warning scores, coma scales, stool charts, levels of care or acuity score, guidelines, checklists—which are used to inform and monitor care and treatment. These are often combined with informal cognitive artefacts including things like the diagnostic rules of thumb used by ear, nose and throat surgeons and found to be responsible for widely different rates of tonsillectomies (Bloor, 1976) (Box 7.6), the 'mindlines' deployed by general practitioners in implementing clinical guidelines (Gabbay and le May, 2004, 2016) (see Box 7.6) and the practices of bricolage of nurses working in general practice settings (Carrier, 2020) (see Box 7.6).

TMT takes seriously the role of artefacts in understanding systems of work. Whether they are formal or informal, material or cognitive, artefacts perform functions in accomplishing a collective activity and have important implications for how action is distributed. Work though Exercise 7.2 before moving to the next domain assumption.

EXERCISE 7.2

Think about a patient from your practice experience and list as many of the artefacts involved in their care.

You can record your answer in the Care Trajectory Management Workbook (see Evolve website).

BOX 7.6 ■ Cognitive Artefacts in Healthcare Practice

Surgeons' Decision-Making Heuristics and the Adenotonsillectomy Enigma

In a classic study in medical sociology, Bloor (1976) used observational methods to examine the decision-making practices of ear, nose and throat surgeons working in the UK National Health Service. He wanted to better understand the well-documented variability in adeno-tonsillectomy rates at this time. Bloor observed 11 surgeons in different outpatient's clinics in the UK as they examined patients. In each case, he produced an analysis of their routine assessment practices—'decision rules' and 'search procedures'. A detailed written report was sent to each surgeon and then discussed at interview to assess the validity of his analyses. He argued that each surgeon used routines consistently in their own practices, but that these routines varied between surgeons. Thus, the statistical patterns were produced by very different 'rules of thumb'—which led some surgeons to advise surgery based on physical findings, and others to weigh up other factors from the patient's medical history which might discourage surgical intervention. Bloor's study predates the rise of evidence-based practice, but even where guidelines and standards exist, doctors use informal mental models—mindlines—to reach decisions in situations of complexity.

Between Guidelines and Mindlines

Gabbay and le May (2004, 2016) have investigated the implementation of guidelines and evidence-based practice in the UK primary care setting. In their initial study they used observational methods to examine how primary care teams put guidelines into practice (2004) with additional data generated from the main study site for a further 5 years. The researchers highlighted the 'remarkable complexity of the context' in which clinical decisions are made. While conceding that the evidence-based practice movement accepts that clinicians should use evidence judiciously in response to the individual circumstances, they note that 'the expected norm of sticking to them with the odd contingent tweak here and there gets nowhere near the challenge of dealing with all the factors that a practitioner needs to weigh up, not as mere occasional add-ons, but as an inherent part of dealing with individual clinical problems' (Gabbay and le May, 2016).

Gabbay and le May argue that in responding to the complexity of decision making, practitioners used 'mindlines'. Mindlines are 'guidelines-in-the-head', in which over a clinical career, a wide range of evidence has been integrated with experiential and tacit knowledge in the clinician's personal guide to practising in varied contexts. Gabbay and le May observed that mindlines were pooled in the workplace, while chatting over coffee, sharing experiences and swapping stories. Through these processes, practitioners were developing collective mindlines for the primary care practice. Gabbay and le May deliberately selected exemplary primary care teams for the purposes of their research, and caution that while this process worked well in the study site, inadequate processes of sharing and modifying mindlines could result in poor practice. Gabbay and le May argue that the processes they observed clearly had an important role in developing mindlines which impact on clinical care, but rather than understanding these practices as obstacles to guideline implementation, there is a need to better understand how they help, and to enable them to flourish through education, training and facilitation.

Bricolage in General Practice Nursing

Carrier (2020) examined how nurses working in primary care used knowledge in their practice. She used ethnographic methods to analyse nurses' work in two primary care settings. Carrier found that while general practice nurses were committed to using evidence together with professional judgment in individualising care to the needs of patients, the social organisation of their work mitigated against the development of collective practice mindlines described by Gabbay and le May (2011). Carrier observed that nurses were prepared to adapt their practice to meet the requirements of the patient, but their knowledge mobilisation strategies were better described as 'bricolage', that is a strategy based on using the resources at hand to deal with the practice situation (Gobbi, 2004), rather than shared mindlines.

Bloor, M., 1976. Bishop Berkeley and the adenotonsillectomy enigma: an exploration of variation in the social construction of medical disposals. Sociology. 10(1), 43–61.

Carrier, J., 2020. An ethnographic exploration of the social organisation of general practice nurses' knowledge use: more than 'mindlines'? J. Res. Nurs. 25(6–7), 604–615. doi: 10.1177/1744987120937411.

Gabbay, J., le May A., 2004. Evidence based guidelines or collectively constructed 'mindlines'? Ethnographic study of knowledge management in primary care. Br. Med. J. 329(7473), 1249–1252.

Gabbay, J., le May, A., 2011. Practice-Based Evidence for Health Care: Clinical Mindlines. Routledge, Abingdon.

Gabbay, J., le May, A., 2016. Mindlines: making sense of evidence in practice. Br. J. Gen. Pract. 66(649), 402–403.

Gobbi, M., 2004. Nursing practice as bricoleur activity: a concept explored. Nurs. Inq. 12(2), 117–125.

DOMAIN ASSUMPTION 4: ACTIVITIES HAVE A SOCIOMATERIAL DISTRIBUTION

The fourth domain assumption of TMT, which is informed by insights from actor network theory (Latour, 1992, 2005) (see Box 7.2), is that activities within a system of work have a sociomaterial distribution; that is, they are shared between people and artefacts. From this perspective, participants do not simply work with artefacts; artefacts are understood as 'acting' within an overall activity. For example, in healthcare systems across the developed world, a preoperative checklist is used to coordinate the preparation of patients for surgery. The checklist directs the user's attention to the existence of allergies, when the patient last ate or drank, their weight and whether they have loose teeth, dental caps or crowns. It does not prompt consideration of the person's social networks, dietary preferences and hobbies or any of the other facets of the person's identity that may be relevant for care. These concerns are simply not relevant for operating theatre work and the checklist excludes them from the information that is required. In the analysis of networks, actor network theory distinguishes between intermediaries and mediators. Intermediaries make no difference to actor networks, whereas mediators shape network relationships and should be the object of study. Returning to the preoperative checklist example, from an actor network theory perspective, the checklist is an actor which *mediates* the work of preparing the patient for their operation. It translates the requirements of the anaesthetist, surgeon and operating department into the practices of ward nurses and junior doctors to ensure that the all the necessary actions have been accomplished to ensure that the patient is acceptable for surgery. It also excludes extraneous information.

All artefacts have distinctive *affordances*, that is, properties that determine how they can be used, what they can do and how they act (Gibson, 1979). Sometimes, artefacts perform functions that might otherwise be performed by a person (this is known as delegation (Latour, 1992)); for example, an electric food mixer does the work of combining the ingredients in a cake, rather than this being performed manually by the cook. Sometimes, artefacts require work from humans to fulfil their functions (this is known as prescription (Latour, 1992)); for example, a door presupposes that human actors will open and shut it, if it is to do the job of closing a hole in the wall (Latour, 1998). These assumptions are built into the artefact, and in actor network theory are referred to as a *script*. The basic point is to understand that activities typically have a sociometrical distribution. Understanding how an activity is distributed and organised between people and the artefacts requires attention to the relationships that are involved (Exercise 7.3).

Knowing that materials and technologies do not simply support activity but transform the task and the distribution of work highlights how the introduction of new technologies has important implications for practice (Box 7.7). Consider the actions involved in writing an essay using a pen and paper compared to those required when using a word processor. Irrespective of an individual's particular approach to writing, the handwritten essay requires rather more preplanning to avoid errors, false starts or unsightly corrections as, unlike a working with a word processor, there is no scope for changes of structure or moving text around once it has been committed to the page. There is also no spell-checker!

EXERCISE 7.3

Consider the use of different artefacts in mediating the work involved in monitoring and recording patient fluid balance. Mrs Barratt-Lee is nil by mouth and has an intravenous infusion and urinary catheter. Mrs Diamond is eating and drinking normally (but requires support with nutrition and hydration) and is not catheterised but experiences occasional urgency of micturition. The aim of the activity is the same—to maintain an accurate record of fluid balance—but the actions required to achieve the aim, and its distribution across human and nonhuman actors, are quite different, with different implications for the work of nurses.

You can record your answer in the Care Trajectory Management Workbook (see Evolve website).

BOX 7.7 ■ Prioritising the Mobilisation of Emergency Medical Services—The Work of Call Operators and Computers at the Healthcare Gateway

As part of a wider research project on care coordination across the healthcare system, I studied the prioritisation and despatch of emergency medical services (EMS) in an ambulance control centre (Allen, 2021). All calls to the EMS were managed by call handlers who worked with a computer-supported prioritisation system: The Medical Priority Dispatch System (MPDS). Formal emergency services prioritisation technologies were adopted in the UK in 1997. These are computerised expert systems characteristically built on abstract universalised rules and algorithms that capture the knowledge and practices required to triage calls in a standardised way. Before this, call handlers would just ask whatever questions they considered relevant to the case, a process that resulted in inconsistency and poor diagnostic accuracy.

Expert systems, like the MPDS, are designed to limit the autonomy of users to ensure consistency and lessen risk. They are an increasingly attractive in the context of fiscal constraint as it enables functions to be undertaken by low-skilled workers. Point-of-contact call handlers in the study site were not clinically qualified, with many coming to the role having worked in telesales and customer services.

The MPDS required call handlers to ask scripted questions in a predetermined order and enter the required caller information into the system. Call handlers could not progress through the system until a question had been answered and the data entered. Compliance with these expectations was routinely monitored. In contrast to other research that has evidenced the skills of users in working flexibly around the constraints of expert systems (Greatbatch et al., 2005; Pope et al., 2013), in this study, call handlers did not operate outside of the technology.

The study revealed the interactional troubles call handlers experienced in working with the prioritisation system and the challenges they encountered in negotiating with callers—many of whom were understandably distressed—to provide the information required to progress through the MPDS. Poor information could result in the MPDS assigning an incorrect priority category to calls. In cases where the call handler was concerned that a call had not been categorised as a sufficiently urgent priority, they would leave their workstation and talk to the despatch operatives who were responsible for allocating EMS resources. While this was a largely informal process, the sensemaking skills of call handlers in detecting inaccurate response categories was recognised by clinical desk staff:

Paramedic: 'They are not clinical and so it is not fair to make judgement calls. But they are very good the call takers. They will come up and say, this has come out as a green 3 – no way! So we had an example of an eight year old child who was having an allergic reaction and the call handler came across to alert me to their concerns with the category. Otherwise if its low on the stack – say green 3 – then you may be three pages back and not necessarily triaged. [...] I had a code which was a child who was very short of breath and had pruritus – they were itching for Wales – and they could still feel the peanut in the back of their throat. There was an APP (Advanced Paramedic Practitioner) around the corner and the first thing they did was to bang them full of adrenalin. And in the words of the APP if the call handler hadn't looked at this then the child would have been dead. He owes his life to a proactive call handler. We all have to work together'. (Field notes)

Allen, D., 2021. Prioritising the mobilisation of emergency medical services: patient making at the healthcare gateway. J. Health Organ. Manag. 35(2), 160–176. doi:10.1108/JHOM-07-2020-0305/full/html.

Greatbatch, D., Hanlon, G., Goode, J., O'Caithain, A., Strangleman, T., Luff, D., 2005. Telephone triage, expert systems and clinical expertise. Sociol. Health Illn. 27(6), 802–830.

Pope, C., Halford, S., Turnball, J., Prichard, J., Calestani, M., May, C., 2013. Using computer decision support systems in NHS emergency and urgent care: ethnographic study using normalisation process theory. BMC Health Serv. Res. 13, 111.

Summary

This chapter has introduced TMT, and its underlying domain assumptions. Taken together the four domain assumptions draw into view the fluidity and sociomaterial complexity of healthcare work and offer a lens through which to comprehend and describe the everyday organisation of patient care. The next chapter will describe and explain the core concepts of TMT which offer a vocabulary through which to articulate how actors work together in accomplishing a shared goal in turbulent conditions.

SUMMARY OF KEY LEARNING

- TMT is a sociological theory which describes the relationships between people, materials and technologies in achieving a goal in dynamic systems of work.
- TMT is founded on four domain assumptions which frame how we see healthcare organisation:
  - An ecological perspective in which the interrelationships between system elements and the wider environment shape activity
  - A process view of organisation which foregrounds the agency of participants in creating order within conditions of stability and fluidity
  - An emphasis on artefacts in systems of work
  - An understanding of the sociomaterial distribution of an activity between people and artefacts and how these impacts on the task at hand.
- Together, the domain assumptions offer a way of understanding healthcare systems for the purposes of trajectory management.

QUICK QUIZ

- What is a grounded theory?
- What is a middle range theory?
- Which two processes are associated with a process view of organisation?
- What is an artefact?
- What is the difference between a formal or an informal artefact?
- What is meant by 'affordance' in descriptions of artefacts?

References

Abbott, A., 1988. The System of Professions: An Essay on the Division of Expert Labor. University of Chicago Press, Chicago, IL.

Allen, D., 2001. The Changing Shape of Nursing Practice: The Role of Nurses in the Hospital Division of Labour. Routledge, London and New York.

Allen, D., 2009. From boundary concept to boundary object: the practice and politics of care pathway development. Soc. Sci. Med. 69 (3), 354–361.

Allen, D., 2015. The Invisible Work of Nurses: Hospitals, Organisation and Healthcare. Routledge, London and New York.

Allen, D., 2018. Translational Mobilisation Theory: a new paradigm from understanding the organisational components of nursing work. Int. J. Nurs. Stud. 79, 36–42.

Allen, D., May, C., 2017. Organizing practice and practicing organization: towards an outline of translational mobilisation theory. Sage Open. doi:10.1177/2158244017707993 April-June, 1-14.

Allen, D., Griffiths, L., Lyne, P., 2004a. Understanding complex trajectories in health and social care provision. Sociol. Health Illn. 26 (7), 1008–1030.

Allen, D., Griffiths, L., Lyne, P., 2004b. Accommodating health and social care need: routine resource alloca-tion processes in stroke rehabilitation. Sociol. Health Illn. 26 (4), 411–432.

Banja, J., 2010. The normalization of deviance in healthcare delivery. Bus. Horiz. 53 (2), 139.

Barach, P, Phelps, G., 2013. Clinical sensemaking: a systematic approach to reduce the impact of normalised deviance in the medical profession. J. R. Soc. Med. 106 (10), 387–390.

Bloor, M., 1976. Bishop Berkeley and the adenotonsillectomy enigma: an exploration of variation in the social construction of medical disposals. Sociology 10 (1), 43–61.

Bourdieu, P., 1977. Outline of a Theory of Practice. Cambridge University Press, Cambridge, UK.

Carrier, J., 2020. An ethnographic exploration of the social organisation of general practice nurses' knowledge use: more than 'mindlines'? J. Res. Nurs 25 (6-7), 604–615. doi:10.1177/1744987120937411.

Engeström, Y., 2000. Activity theory as a framework for analysing and redesigning work. Ergonomics 43, 960–972.

Fligstein, N., McAdam, D., 2011. Toward a general theory of strategic action fields. Sociol. Theory 29, 1–26.

Freidson, E., 1976. The division of labour as social interaction. Soc. Probl. 23, 304–313.

Gabbay, J., le May, A., 2004. Evidence based guidelines or collectively constructed 'mindlines'? Ethnographic study of knowledge management in primary care. Br. Med. J. 329 (7473), 1249–1252.

Gabbay, J., le May, A., 2016. Mindlines: making sense of evidence in practice. Br. J. of Gen. Pract. 66 (649), 402–403.

Garfinkel, H., 1967. Studies in Ethnomethodology. Prentice Hall, Englewood Cliffs, NJ.

Gibson, JJ., 1979. The Ecological Approach to Visual Perception. Taylor & Francis, Boulder, CO.

Giddens, A., 1984. The Constitution of Society: Outline of a Theory of Structuration. Polity Press, Cambridge, UK.

Glaser, BG, Strauss, AL., 1965. Awareness of Dying. Aldine Transaction, New Brunswick, NJ.

Glaser, BG., Strauss, AL., 1967. The Discovery of Grounded Theory: Strategies for Qualitative Research. Aldine Publishing Company, Chicago, IL.

Hardey, M., Payne, S., Coleman, P., 2000. Scraps: hidden nursing information and its influence on the delivery of care. J. Adv. Nurs. 32, 208–214.

Hernes, T., 2014. A Process Theory of Organization. Oxford University Press, Oxford.

Hughes, EC., 1984. The Sociological Eye: Selected Papers. Transaction Books. New Brunswick, NJ, and London.

Latour, B., 1992. Where are the missing masses? The sociology of a few mundane artifacts. In: Bijker, WE., Law, J. (Eds.), Shaping Technology/Building Society: Studies in Sociotechnical Change. MIT Press, Cambridge, MA, pp. 225–258.

Latour, B., 1998. Mixing humans and nonhumans together: the sociology of a door closer. In: Star, SL. (Ed.), Ecologies of Knowledge: Work and Politics in Science and Technology. State University New York Press, New York, pp. 257–277.

Latour, B., 2005. Reassembling the Social: An Introduction to Actor-Network-Theory. Oxford University Press, Oxford.

Leary, A., Bushe, D., Oldman, C., Lawler, J., Punshon, G., 2021. A thematic analysis of the prevention of future deaths reports in healthcare from HM coroners in England and Wales 2016–2019. J. Patient Saf. Risk Manag. 26 (1), 14–21. doi:10.1177/2516043521992651.

May, C., Finch, T., 2009. Implementing, embedding and integration: an outline of normalization process theory. Sociology 43 (3), 535–554.

May, CR., Eton, DT., Boehmer, K., Gallacher, K., Hunt, K., Macdonald, S., et al., 2014. Rethinking the patient: using Burden of Treatment Theory to understand the changing dynamics of illness. BMC Health Serv. Res. 14, 281. doi:10.1186/1472-6963-14-281.

Nicolini, D., 2012. Practice Theory, Work, and Organization: An Introduction. Oxford University Press, Oxford.

Strauss, A., Schatzman, I., Bucher, R., Ehrlich, D., Sabshin, M., 1963. The hospital and its negotiated order. In: Freidson, E. (Ed.), The Hospital in Modern Society. Free Press, New York, pp. 147–169.

Strauss, AL., Schatzman, L., Bucher, R., Ehrlich, D., Sabshin, M., 1964. Psychiatric Ideologies and Institu-tions. The Free Press of Glencoe Collier-Macmillan, London.

Strauss, A., Fagerhaugh, S., Suczet, B., Wiener, C., 1985. Social Organization of Medical Work. University of Chicago Press, Chicago, IL.

Talamo, A., Mellini, B., Barbieri, B., 2017. The role of locally-designed organizational artifacts in support-ing nurses' work: an ethnographic study on the wards. Professioni Infermieristiche 70 (2), 115–125. doi:10.7429/pi.2017.702115.

Timmermans, S., Berg, M., 2003. The Gold Standard: The Challenge of Evidence-based Medicine and Standardization in Health Care. Temple University Press, Philadelphia, PA.

Weick, KE., 1969. The Social Psychology of Organizing. Random House, London.

Suggested Reading

The Sociomaterial Distribution of Work

Allen, D., 2016. The importance, challenges, and prospects of taking work practices into account for healthcare quality improvement: nursing work and patient status at a glance white boards. J. Health. Organ. Manag. 30 (4), 672–689.
This paper draws on data from *The Invisible Work of Nurses* (Allen, 2015) to highlight the limitations of substituting people with inanimate technologies for the purposes of coordinating patient care. It contributes to critical debates about whether lean management techniques make nursing and healthcare work more efficient and release time for nursing care.

Donetto, S., Desai, A., Zoccatelli, G., Allen, D., Brearley, S., Rafferty, AM., Robert, G., 2021. Patient experience data as enacted: sociomaterial perspectives and 'singular-multiples' in health care quality improvement research. Sociol. Health Illn. 43 (4), 1032–1050, doi:10.1111/1467-9566.13276.
This paper draws on actor network theory to explore how patient experience data 'acts' for the purposes of quality improvement. While illustrating how patient experience data participated in quality improvement processes, the study also shows how patient experienced data acted in different ways and with a range of effects depending on the network of relationships in which it was enrolled. By showing the relationships through which quality improvement is achieved or not, the study opens the possibility for thinking about how things can be done differently. The research involved workshops with the study sites, and preliminary sharing of the study findings highlighted that organisations could envisage practical changes to how they operated in order that data were deployed and put to work to best effect.

CHAPTER 8

Conceptualising Healthcare Work for Care Trajectory Management

LEARNING OUTCOMES

At the end of this chapter, you will be able to:
- Describe the core components of Translational Mobilisation Theory
- Combine this learning with your understanding of the domain assumptions of Translational Mobilisation Theory
- Apply Translational Mobilisation Theory to healthcare

Introduction

Having described and explained the domain assumptions of Translational Mobilisation Theory (TMT) and their implications for seeing and understanding the organisation of healthcare, this chapter explores the core components of the theory. Together, these form a framework for thinking systematically about the 'what, where and how' of accomplishing a shared goal, that is grounded in the material and cognitive practices and relational mechanisms that support or inhibit concerted action (Allen, 2016). Developing this kind of granular understanding of an activity is important for several purposes. For research, it allows for comparison across different settings and fosters the opportunity for cross-sector learning. For quality improvement, it facilitates understanding of the sociomaterial processes a new intervention it is designed to improve, that is, the work-as-done. For our purposes, it lays the ground for explaining and describing the mechanisms and practices of care trajectory management.

The Core Components of Translational Mobilisation Theory

TMT has three core components which build on its domain assumptions. The *project* refers to the collective activity or shared goal. The *strategic action field* refers to the context in which a project

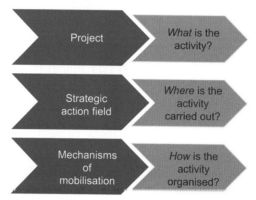

Fig. 8.1   Translational Mobilisation Theory—core components.

of collective activity is carried out which creates the conditions that shape action. The *mechanisms* refer to how the project activity is organised (Fig. 8.1).

Together, these components create a structure for the systematic analysis of how collective action is organised in unpredictable work environments wherever these are found.

Projects: Defining the Activity of Interest

Projects are the primary focus of attention in TMT and define the activity of interest. A project refers to the ecological (see Chapter 7, Box 7.2) arrangement of people, technologies and artefacts involved in collective action oriented to a shared goal. Projects follow a trajectory in time and space. They have a beginning, a middle and an end; they take place in a particular context, involve key interventions and events and have distinctive sociomaterial relationships. Defining the project sets the boundaries around the activity and focuses attention on the relationships of interest. So, in applying the theory to healthcare, the project could refer to the totality of a patient's hospital care, or the ongoing management of a long-term condition, or it could be more narrowly focused on a particular process within an overall trajectory of care—such as a clinical procedure or discharge planning. An alternative strategy is to take an individual actor (remember this can be human and nonhuman)—such as an observation chart or an occupational role—and consider the wider project of activity in which it is located. This kind of approach is helpful for quality improvement purposes in appraising how the introduction of a new technology might impact on practice or to highlight necessary revisions in documents or forms to enable them to better fulfil their functions.

For illustrative purposes, this chapter deploys patient rescue trajectories as the project of interest. A rescue trajectory refers to the actions that are necessary to detect and act on signs of deterioration in a hospitalised patient. Deterioration is often preceded by a period of physiological instability which, when recognised, provides an opportunity for earlier intervention, and improved outcome. Ensuring that staff recognise, relay and react to signs of deterioration requires coordination and collaboration across professional and departmental boundaries in conditions of uncertainty and involves the use of a range of technologies and artefacts (Burke et al., 2020). In broad terms the elements involved in rescue trajectories include the patient, family (a parent in the case of children), ward staff (healthcare support staff, nurses, doctors), emergency response team, critical care staff (intensivists, outreach teams), monitoring technologies, observation charts, early warning scores or indicators and escalation policies. The precise combination of elements and their relationships will be shaped by the conditions in the local context, which is why understanding the strategic action field has value. Before moving to the next section, complete Exercise 8.1. This is the first of 10 exercises in this chapter that are designed to support the application of TMT to an activity of your choice.

Select an activity with which you have experience. This can be an example from healthcare, but an activity from another context you are familiar with can be used for this exercise. Just make sure it is an activity that is dependent on collective effort, that is, people working together.

First, define the scope of the activity.

Second, list all the people, materials and technologies that are involved in the activity.

You can record your answer in the Care Trajectory Management Workbook (see Evolve website).

Strategic Action Field: Where Does the Activity Take Place?

The strategic action field is the second core component of TMT. This concept is drawn from the work of Fligstein and McAdam (2011) (see Chapter 7, Box 7.2). It refers to the setting in which the project takes place and focuses on the features of the environment which condition how an activity is accomplished. These contextual features are important to understand. Healthcare environments are highly variable, and such differences have important implications for the organisation of work. There are huge disparities globally between developed and developing countries, which impact on not only how projects of collective action are organised but also which projects are important. Even within a single healthcare system, there are clear differences between the acute hospital, home care and community contexts, and further differences again within these broad distinctions which shape how work is done. TMT attends to these local environmental conditions through a focus on four salient features of strategic action fields:

- Structures—formal fixed points and positions
- Organising logics—norms, priorities and values that drive action
- Interpretative repertoires—meaning making resources
- Materials—physical infrastructure, technologies and facilities

STRUCTURES

Structures refers to the patterned elements of a strategic action field that generate the entities, positions and relationships through which an activity is organised. While people may come and go, structures are the fixed points in organisations that enable participants to make sense of and order their activity. They include professions, roles, organisations, departments, teams and hierarchies. Although TMT is founded on a process view of organisation, and so does not regard structures as determining activity directly, it recognises that organisational processes are not totally unbridled and that structures condition the possibilities for action. In other words, it matters whether you are a nurse or a physiotherapist, whether you are a junior or a senior team member, and which department or service you work in, even if everyday activity is more fluid than role descriptions and the formal organisational chart suggest.

In the example of a rescue trajectory, TMT draws attention to several salient structures that impact on how activity is organised. The division of labour between nursing and support staff is one important consideration. In some contexts, for example, healthcare support workers are responsible for undertaking monitoring activity, whereas in others, this is a nursing responsibility. This allocation of roles and responsibilities will in turn impact on the policies that are required to ensure signs of deterioration are recognised and acted on. For example, do support staff have a licence to contact medical staff directly if they are concerned, or is there a requirement for this to be mediated through a nurse? A further structural feature of central importance in the functioning of rescue trajectories is the interprofessional relationships between nursing and medicine. There is considerable research evidence that indicates that initiating action across professional boundaries is critical for timely intervention, but it is known to be challenging (Andrews and Waterman, 2005). Nurses report difficulties in persuading doctors to act on their concerns, and doctors express frustration that they do not receive the clinical information required for medical decision-making. Beyond interprofessional relationships, rescue trajectories are also shaped by how care is organised across the key functional units

EXERCISE 8.2

> Return to your project of action and document the structures involved. Here are some prompts to
> assist your thinking:
>   Where do project activities take place?
>   What are the fixed points in the strategic action field?
>   What organisations, departments, teams, roles, professions, actors are involved?
>   Who/what are the primary actors? Where is power located?
>   Which are critical junctures and dependency relationships between actors and actions?
>   What are the key interfaces between collaborators?
>   You can record your answer in the Care Trajectory Management Workbook (see Evolve website).

in a strategic action field: the ward and high-dependency and intensive care units; the emergency
response team if there is one; and the relationships between different departments. Decision-making
about the escalation of care and treatment is influenced by interaction across these organisational
interfaces (Cioffi, 2000). Apply these insights to your own example by completing Exercise 8.2.

ORGANISING LOGICS

Organising logics refer to those elements of a strategic action field—norms, values, priorities—that drive
how things are done in a project of action and shape its purpose. Organising logics are an example of
the institutional logics you learnt about in Chapter 3 (see Complexity 6: Healthcare Is Characterised
by Multiple Institutional Logics). While at one level the higher-order aim of a rescue trajectory should
be the same in any organisation—to recognise, relay and react to signs of deterioration—this may be
mediated by the local conditions in a strategic action field. For example, the drivers for action and
organisational logics in a tertiary hospital with intensive care and high-dependency units will be subtly
different from those of a smaller hospital without such facilities and where escalation of care entails
transferring patients to a geographically distant specialist facility. Professionals in a tertiary hospital
may be more prepared to wait before acting to move a patient to intensive care, whereas this could be
a high-risk strategy in hospitals where transfers cannot be organised as swiftly and where delays could
be consequential for the care or treatment of the patient. As described in Chapter 3, organisations
are shaped by multiple and sometimes competing logics. While the safety logic is the dominant logic
informing rescue trajectories, this can be impacted and disrupted by the intersection of other logics
to the detriment of patient care. For example, research has shown that junior doctors can be deterred
from escalating care if they fear professional censure from senior medical staff if their concerns prove
to be unfounded. Recognition of the dangers of this contradictory logic on rescue trajectories has led
to the call for inculcating a 'no false alarms' culture in systems for detecting and acting on deterioration
(Bonafide et al., 2013; Chua et al., 2013; Entwistle, 2004; Pattison and Eastham, 2012). What are the
logics that influence collective activity in your own example (Exercise 8.3)?

INTERPRETATIVE REPERTOIRES

Interpretative repertoires refer to the formal and informal cognitive artefacts and meaning making
resources available within a strategic action field (see Chapter 7: Domain Assumption 3: Activity Is
Mediated by Artefacts). In the management of rescue trajectories, there is growing use of early warning
scores and track and trigger tools to make sense of signs of deterioration. Track and trigger tools are
formal artefacts that consist of sequential physiological, clinical and observational data recorded and
accumulated on a chart (either paper or digital). When a certain score (achieved by weighting and aggre-
gating each observation) or trigger (observations moving beyond prespecified parameters) is reached,
then an escalation response is initiated (Roland et al., 2014). By specifying physiological thresholds that
indicate deterioration, track and trigger tools take knowledge to the bedside and act as prompts for the
initiation of action (Andrews and Waterman, 2005; Endacott and Westley, 2006). Yet, while track and

EXERCISE 8.3

Document the organising logics involved in your selected project of action; remember that these may be contradictory. Here are some prompts to assist your thinking:

What is the primary driver of activity in the project?

What are the logics that inform the actions of project participants? These can be official or unofficial.

Are there conflicts or ambiguities in the project? What may be the cause of these?

How are accommodations achieved between different logics?

You can record your answer in the Care Trajectory Management Workbook (see Evolve website).

trigger tools can lead to improved detection of deterioration (Lydon et al., 2016; Sønning et al., 2017), there is evidence that rationalising processes using physiological parameters diminishes the importance of other interpretative repertoires within the field which have value in detecting deterioration, such as professional pattern recognition and expert patient or carer knowledge (Box 8.1). In response to this unintended consequence, a growing number of early warning systems now include nonphysiological indicators—such as 'staff concern' or 'parental concern'—as part of the formal artefact (Cioffi, 2000; Mackintosh et al., 2014; McDonnell et al., 2013) and some use formal categorisation processes to identify those patients whom staff have a gut feeling are at risk of deteriorating (Goldenhar et al., 2013) (see Chapter 7: Domain Assumption 4: Activities Have a Sociomaterial Distribution) (Exercise 8.4).

EXERCISE 8.4

List the formal and informal interpretative repertoires involved in your project and how these shape how the activity is accomplished. Here are some prompts to assist your thinking:

What information and knowledge sources are involved in the project? How reliable, accessible and comprehensive are the information sources? Who is responsible for generating the information sources?

What are the formal artefacts and interpretative resources involved in the project? (Polices, risk assessments, guidelines, systems of categorisation, methods or triage processes)

Are informal processes involved?

What is the relationship between available interpretative repertoires?

How do interpretative repertoires in the strategic action field influence how action is organised and with what effect?

You can record your answer in the Care Trajectory Management Workbook (see Evolve website).

BOX 8.1 ■ Formal and Informal Interpretative Repertoires in Rapid Response Systems

Mackintosh et al. (2012) carried out comparative case studies of the rapid response systems in two hospitals using ethnographic methods. Data included 150 hours of observations of ward work, shadowing medical staff and 35 interviews with nurses, doctors, healthcare assistants, safety leads and managers from the wards and in critical care.

Both hospitals included a track and trigger tool and escalation policy as part of the rapid response system. The researchers found that the rapid response system reduced the variability in recording, recognition and response behaviour; formalised understandings of deterioration; and provided a mandate for escalating care across professional and hierarchical boundaries. Introduction of the rapid response system appeared to legitimate the delegation of monitoring activity to healthcare assistants. Markers of deterioration not included in formal risk scores were marginalised and this made it more difficult for staff to escalate case without the 'objective evidence' provided by the score.

Mackintosh, N., Rainey, H., Sandall, J., 2012. Understanding how rapid response systems may improve safety for the acutely ill patient: learning from the frontline. BMJ Qual. Saf. 21(2), 135–144. doi: 10.1136/bmjqs-2011-000147.

MATERIALS

TMT draws attention to the available *materials* in a strategic action field. In this context, materials refer to the physical infrastructure, technologies and concrete resources within a strategic action field, and how these condition the performance of an activity and the sociomaterial distribution of work. In the example of rescue trajectories, relevant materials and technologies include monitoring equipment, technologies for intervening in care and treatment, methods for accumulating and displaying vital signs information and the materials and expertise associated with the ward, emergency response team and high-dependency and intensive care units. Different healthcare contexts give rise to distinctive material arrangements and these influence rescue trajectories in significant ways, place different demands on users and shape the distribution of action (Box 8.2). Consider, for example, the implications for nursing work of continuous electronic patient monitoring systems with automated alerts and alarms, compared with intermittent manual systems that require vital

---

BOX 8.2 ■ Material Insights From the PUMA Study

In the PUMA study (Allen et al., 2022a, 2022b), we developed, implemented and evaluated a novel paediatric early warning system improvement programme. The research was carried out in four hospitals. Quantitative data were collected on clinical outcomes (adverse events) and qualitative data were generated on the paediatric early warning systems in four wards before and after implementation of the intervention. The improvement programme supported clinical teams to assess their practices against the PUMA Standard, an evidence-based model of the core components of an early warning system (Jacob et al., 2019). When each hospital assessed their existing paediatric early warning systems as part of the improvement programme, several identified that a major weakness in the local arrangements for detecting deterioration was a lack of appropriate functioning monitoring equipment. This was a system weakness that was quickly addressed in each site, through purchasing new equipment and putting in place a regular equipment audit.

Over the lifetime of the study, one of the hospitals implemented an electronic early warning system, which was designed to replicate the paper chart staff had worked with previously. Monitoring continued to be manual, but there was now a computerised system for recording vital signs, as well as updating all notes, test results, medication and other information. The electronic system automatically calculated the score for the patient. Implementation of the new system caused several problems for nurses. First, staff expressed concern about the accuracy of the automated scores, which tended to be lower than the paper version. These assumed incorrect scores created an additional step in nurses' monitoring tasks, as they had to manually make a note of what the correct score should be. The new technology also disrupted nursing workflow, as there were often insufficient computers available to allow nurses to enter vital signs data, leading to a delay between monitoring and recording activity, with attendant risks to patient safety, not least as scores were recorded on scraps of paper. Doctors, on the other hand, did not report problems with the technology. Indeed, the implementation of the electronic system enabled doctors to access patient data remotely, which was particularly useful when they were working off the ward. The senior clinicians who led implementation of the electronic system were completely unaware of its impact on nursing work, until we fed this back through the research.

Allen, D., Lloyd, A., Edwards, D., Grant, A., Hood, K., Huang, C., et al., 2022a. Development, implementation and evaluation of an early warning system improvement programme for children in hospital: the PUMA mixed-methods study. Health Soc. Care Deliv. Res. 10(1). doi:10.3310/CHCK4556.

Allen, D., Lloyd, A. Edwards, D., Hood, K., Chao, H., Hughes, J., et al., 2022b. Development, implementation and evaluation of an evidence-based paediatric early warning system improvement programme: the PUMA mixed methods study. BMC Health Serv. Res. 22(1), 9.

Jacob, N., Moriarty, Y., Lloyd, A., Mann, M., Tume, LN., Sefton, G., et al., 2019. Optimising paediatric afferent component early warning systems: a hermeneutic systematic literature review and model development. BMJ Paediatr. Open. 9(11), e028796. doi:10.1136/bmjopen-2018-028796.

EXERCISE 8.5

Document the infrastructure, technologies and materials involved in your project of interest. Remember, these can be formal or informal. Here are some prompts to assist your thinking:

What material artefacts are involved in the activity?

What technologies are involved in the activity?

How is the activity impacted by the physical infrastructure in the strategic action field?

How is work distributed between people and technologies and with what effects?

You can record your answer in the Care Trajectory Management Workbook (see Evolve website).

signs to be measured, recorded and a score calculated by the bedside carer to determine the level of risk and signal a warning alert. Examine the materials involved in your own project example, and complete Exercise 8.5.

Mechanisms of Mobilisation: How Is Collective Action Accomplished?

Mechanisms are the third core component of TMT. Mechanisms describe and explain *how* the goals of a project are accomplished. TMT specifies five mechanisms through which collective action is organised:

- Object formation—how participants in a project create the objects of their practice
- Translation—how practice objects are shared, and differing viewpoints accommodated
- Articulation—how the elements of a project are assembled, aligned and mobilised
- Reflexive monitoring—how oversight of a project is achieved
- Sensemaking—how project participants produce meaning and create order

OBJECT FORMATION

Object formation is the first mechanism in TMT; it refers to the processes through which participants involved in a project use the interpretative and material resources within a strategic action field to create the objects of their practice. 'Patients' are the objects of practice in healthcare. While this may be a very different, and potentially uncomfortable, way of thinking about professional work, it highlights the fact that when people arrive in healthcare systems in need of care and treatment, action must be taken to enable them to become the focus of professional attention.

Applied to healthcare, the concept of object formation refers to how people with problems and concerns are transformed into 'patients' by healthcare workers. Attending to mechanisms of object formation draws into view the multiple versions of the patient that are produced as people are understood by different participants for different purposes. While all members of the multidisciplinary team are patient focused, broadly speaking, professions and specialisms each create their own singular understandings of the person as a patient to guide their practice. Nurses assess for nursing care needs, doctors assess for medical needs, and allied health professionals assess needs for rehabilitation and assistive technologies. Patients express frustration about having to retell their stories and histories, but in each case the healthcare professional brings a singular set of cognitive and practical concerns to the interaction. The result is that as objects of healthcare practice (aka patients), people are understood and 'seen' in numerous ways for different purposes. You may wish to revisit the discussion on professional vision in thinking about this point (see Chapter 1, Making the Invisible, Visible: Why Concepts Matter for Nursing Practice).

In *The Body Multiple*, Anne-Marie Mol (2002) traces the numerous enactments of the patient through which a diagnosis of atherosclerosis is reached. She shows how the 'atherosclerosis'

EXERCISE 8.6

Document the objects of practice involved in your project of interest. Here are some prompts to assist your thinking:

What are the moments of object formation?

Who are the agents involved? What is the purpose of their practice?

What artefacts are involved? What are the objects of practice that emerge from these processes? What are their interrelationships?

How are objects of practice distributed in time and space?

You can record your answer in the Care Trajectory Management Workbook (see Evolve website).

observed in the clinic differs from the 'atherosclerosis' that is created by the vascular laboratory, which diverges from the 'atherosclerosis' generated in the operating theatre. Mol (1999) suggests that if we accept that reality is performed differently through a variety of practices, then there may be choices about which versions of an object is to prevail. This, she argues, requires us to consider where such options are located and what is at stake when a decision must be taken between alternative versions (see also Latimer, 2000). We saw this in the example of Edward Murphy (see Case Study 7.1) in Chapter 7, in which the various perspectives of health and social care professions produced a different framing of Edward, his family and the discharge problem. Edward was an exceptional case, but it should not detract from the main point here, which is that in healthcare practice, in an individual case, there are multiple versions of the person as 'patient' in circulation. A major challenge for care coordination is how these diverse understandings can be brought together to enable concerted action.

If we drill down into our rescue trajectory example, we can identify multiple examples of object formation. First, an individual must be identified as at risk of deterioration and a regime of vital signs monitoring instigated. In most healthcare settings, all patients will be monitored as a matter of routine, but the frequency of observations is informed by an assessment of risk, which constructs the person as a particular kind of patient, who has the potential to become critically unwell. Second, vital signs tracking can lead to further object formation, by triggering an early warning score, which indicates that the patient's physiological status is a cause for concern and requires action of some kind. Third, staff may designate a patient a 'watcher' based on clinical intuition or parental concern in the case of children. The watcher status is a safety intervention used to identify those patients the clinical team consider may be at risk of becoming sicker. Finally, having identified the patient to be at risk, further object formation will occur by matching the issues of concern to a specific intervention, namely, does the patient need to be seen by a doctor, do they require treatment, do they need to be transferred to intensive care. Of course, these designations of the patient relate only to the rescue trajectory; over the course of an admission to hospital, a whole host of other understandings of the person, as patient, will be generated by those involved in their care and treatment. For our purposes, however, the notion of object formation draws into view how, in the case of rescue trajectories, the patient is made and remade for the purposes of mobilising their care. How does the mechanism of object formation relate to your project example (Exercise 8.6)?

TRANSLATION

Translation is the second mechanism in TMT. Derived from actor network theory (Latour, 2005) (see Chapter 7, Box 7.2), translation refers to the processes that enable practice objects to be shared between participants and these different understandings accommodated. Returning to our rescue trajectory example, it points to the actions necessary for a patient who is an object of concern for nursing staff ('nurse worried') to be translated into a clinical priority for the doctor and, if necessary, translated into the focus of intervention by the emergency response team. Even when deterioration is identified, mobilising action across professional boundaries can be challenging, with differences in language between doctors and nurses and power dynamics contributory factors (Mackintosh and Sandall, 2010). In some contexts where there is a stable healthcare team and strong interprofessional working, translational processes may be accomplished through everyday mechanisms of communication. However, in other cases, the use of structured communication tools—early warning score, SBAR (Box 8.3)—can be more effective. Structured communication tools mediate action: by transforming a series of discrete observations into a summative indicator of deterioration, tools package the patient's status into a form that can be readily communicated (Andrews and Waterman, 2005) and can be effective in overcoming professional hierarchies and cultural differences (Box 8.4). Before reading further, complete Exercise 8.7.

BOX 8.3 ■ **Definition: SBAR**

SBAR is an acronym for Situation, Background, Assessment, Recommendation. It is a structured communication technique that provides a framework for communicating in healthcare.

BOX 8.4 ■ **The Use of Early Warning Scores as a Translation Device**

Andrews and Waterman (2005) report on a grounded theory study of how nurses report physiological deterioration effectively. The paper draws on a wider qualitative research project which used interviews and observations to examine the practical problems faced by nurses in detecting physiological deterioration. The authors observe that signs of deterioration are often subtle and identified by nurses deploying intuitive knowledge. The challenge is to package this information and present evidence of physiological deterioration in a format that mobilises doctors to act. Doctors, like nurses, must manage their workload, and quantifiable data enable them to make judgements about a patient's condition and how urgently the patient needs to be seen. The authors argue that the early warning score facilitates this decision-making as it packages information on vital signs together so that an assessment can be made as to why a patient is scoring. Subtle changes in patients are difficult to articulate and not all nurses in the study were confident in using medical terminology. The authors found that the early warning score gave nurses a concise and unambiguous means of communicating deterioration to medical staff. The authors argue that the early warning score is as important for the purposes of communication as it is about detecting deterioration.

Andrews, T., Waterman, H., 2005. Packaging: a grounded theory of how to report physiological deterioration effectively. J. Adv. Nurs. 52(5), 473–481.

EXERCISE 8.7

Return to your project of interest and think about the translations that are necessary to enable participants to work together to accomplish the activity. These might not be linear processes as in the example of rescue trajectories; concentrate on key moments of communication between participants when one participant's interpretation and way of describing a situation needs to be translated into the language of another to facilitate understanding or mobilise action. Here are some prompts to assist your thinking:

Where are the occasions when translational action is required?
Who is involved?
What is involved?
Whose perspectives need to be considered for collective action to proceed?
You can record your answer in the Care Trajectory Management Workbook (see Evolve website).

EXERCISE 8.8

Returning to your project of interest, think about those aspects of the activity that need to be articulated and how this happens. What are the formal or informal mechanisms involved? Here are some prompts to assist your thinking:

What are the elements (activities, materials) in the activity that need to be aligned?
How is articulation work organised?
Are there formal processes?
Is someone formally responsible for the articulation of an activity?
Is articulation informal?
Who does informal articulation work? When does it take place?
What are the materials, technologies and interpretative repertoires that support articulation work?

You can record your answer in the Care Trajectory Management Workbook (see Evolve website).

ARTICULATION

The third mechanism in TMT is *articulation*. Strauss et al. (1985) developed the concept of articulation to refer to the work that is necessary in managing the relationship between contingency and control in healthcare work. Articulate comes from *articulus*, the Latin term for small joint, and it refers to the act of connecting things together to allow movement. The authors adopt this expression in preference to the more conventional language of coordination, as the latter term presupposes planning and control, and their aim was to draw attention to the multiplicity of both formal and informal interventions required to hold things together in situations of emergent organisation. As outlined in Chapters 3 and 4, for a whole range of reasons, much of patient care challenges notions of rational–linear organisation and management as this is conventionally understood. Having developed the concept of articulation in the healthcare context, the authors extended its application to refer to the full spectrum of work processes necessary to align the actions, knowledge and resources in projects of collective action and ensure that 'the staff's collective efforts add up to more than discrete and conflicting bits of accomplished work' (Strauss et al., 1985, p. 151).

Articulation can be thought of as a kind of 'supra work'; it requires skills and resources over and above the immediate task at hand. In other words, it is the work that makes the work, work, and as such it is an essential element in emergent organisation. Healthcare systems often have well-specified and routinised arrangements for time-critical interventions, but these are not available for all eventualities and other actions are necessary to ensure the elements in a project of action are aligned as and when they are required. Moreover, the success of even the most formalised processes depends on management and tinkering around the edges. For example, in rescue trajectories, hospitals normally have in place formal escalation policies which specify the order of actions to be taken in different scenarios, but in practice, these require negotiations and adjustments to ensure all the elements are in place to support action. Work through Exercise 8.8 and consider how mechanisms of articulation are relevant to your own project.

REFLEXIVE MONITORING

The fourth mechanism in TMT is *reflexive monitoring*. Derived from research on implementation (May and Finch, 2009), reflexive monitoring refers to the processes through which actors collectively or individually appraise and review the progress of an activity. In a distributed field of action such as healthcare (see Chapter 3: Complexity 3: Healthcare Is Distributed Work), reflexive monitoring is the means through which members accomplish situational awareness (Gilson, 1995). Situational awareness can refer to the awareness of an individual, a team or a system (Endsley, 1995), and there are a whole range of mechanisms through which it can be achieved that are conditioned by the wider strategic action field. In our rescue trajectory example, several hospitals in the PUMA (The Paediatric early warning system Utilisation and Morbidity Avoidance) study (see Box 8.2) introduced mechanisms to

> **BOX 8.5 ■ Reflexive Monitoring and Situational Awareness in Delivery Suites**
>
> Mackintosh et al. (2009) carried out a qualitative study of arrangements for ensuring team situational awareness in the delivery suites in four purposively selected English hospitals. Data were collected through observations of practice and conversations with staff while they worked. In all four sites, the key elements for supporting team situational awareness included a whiteboard, handover and a delivery suite coordinator. These were supplemented by other supports which included ongoing communication between teams, ward clerks who had knowledge of room occupancy and written notices. Primary and supplementary arrangements were perceived to complement and compensate for each other.
>
> The authors observed that it was the interplay of each element in these arrangements that facilitated high levels of team situation awareness. In an ideal configuration, the whiteboard, coordinator and handover were used across the team to accumulate and share information. The whiteboard was clear and regularly updated, the handover was attended by all the team, and the coordinator did not carry a client so that they could support other staff. At the other end of the spectrum, the principal elements in the arrangements were compromised: the whiteboard was small and not regularly updated, team handovers were insufficiently inclusive and/or not prioritised, and the coordinator was not accessible and had responsibility for clients. In such circumstances, staff had greater reliance on supplementary supports to maintain awareness of the delivery suite activity. The study is a powerful illustration of why it is essential that interventions are appropriately embedded in practice to be effective in generating the mechanisms necessary to support health care quality and safety.
>
> ---
>
> Mackintosh, N., Berridge, EJ., Freeth, D., 2009. Supporting structures for team situation awareness and decision making: insights from delivery suites. J. Eval. Clin. Pract. 15, 46–54.

EXERCISE 8.9

What are the processes through which participants monitor the status of activities in your project of interest? Once again, this can be formal or informal, and it can be at individual, team or system level, or include elements of each. Here are some prompts to assist your thinking.

What are the formal and informal mechanisms of reflexive monitoring?
What materials, technologies and interpretative resources are involved?
How intense are reflexive monitoring processes?
How is reflexive monitoring work distributed?
What are the challenges involved in maintaining an overview of the activity?
What are the consequences of not having an overview of activities?
You can record your answer in the Care Trajectory Management Workbook (see Evolve website).

increase team situational awareness as part of their system improvement programme. These included the introduction of safety huddles—a short multidisciplinary meeting focused on the patients of concern; whiteboards which displayed patient information, including at-risk status; and arrangements to ensure information sharing between the nursing and medical handovers (Allen et al., 2022a, 2022b). The interventions were designed to ensure that all members of the team had a common understanding of the patients at risk and were appraised of the plan of action in the event of deterioration. Research by Mackintosh et al. highlights that multiple strategies working in concert maximise situational awareness (Box 8.5). What is the role of reflexive monitoring in your example project (Exercise 8.9)?

SENSEMAKING

The final mechanism in TMT is *sensemaking*. Derived from the work of the social psychologist Karl Weick (1969, 1995), sensemaking refers to the processes and practical activities through which actors interpret and create order in conditions of complexity. In a process view of organisation, it is the mechanism that connects organisational structures with the fluidity of everyday practice, such that 'sensemaking and organization constitute one another' (Weick, 1995, p. 410). From this perspective, then, organisational structures, routines and procedures are the practical resources through which actors interpret and enact the social world. It is not formal structures that determine action, rather stability emerges from the organising and sensemaking activity of participants (Hernes and Maitlis, 2010).

So how does sensemaking apply to rescue trajectories? Answering this question draws attention to how staff reach a decision on the appropriate action within the formal processes in place for that purpose. This involves interpreting vital signs data and formal track and trigger tools, taking account of the perspectives of the patient and family, and deploying professional judgement to act on these data in ways which can be accounted for within organisational structures and processes. The relationship between formal structures and everyday sensemaking practice was thrown into sharp relief in one hospital in the PUMA study, where we observed that expert nurses modified the paediatric early warning track and trigger tool if the score generated did not coincide with their intuition about the status of the patient. While the track and trigger tool in this site did not include a score which reflected nurses' concerns, it did include a section for 'parental concern'. If nurses were concerned about the patient, they would use the 'parental concern' function to generate a score that justified escalation of care to medical staff (irrespective of whether parents had expressed concerns or not). There is a growing body of evidence which points to the importance of combining formalised systems with the judgements of healthcare professionals in optimising rescue trajectories (Box 8.6). Consider the role of sensemaking in your own project by completing Exercise 8.10.

> **BOX 8.6** ■ **The Mechanisms by Which Early Warning Scores Impact Patient Safety**
>
> Bonafide et al. (2013) report on a qualitative study of the use of early warning scores (EWSs) in the paediatric context. Data were generated through 57 semistructured interviews with doctors and nurses who had recently cared for patients with score failures. There were four main findings.
>
> First, participants indicated that the EWS alerted physicians and nurses to concerning changes and prompted them to think critically about deterioration.
>
> *Sometimes I feel like if you want things to be okay you can kind of write them off, but when you have to write [the EWS] down…it kind of jogs you to think, maybe something is going on or maybe someone else needs to know about this.*
>
> Second, the EWS provided less experienced nurses with vital sign reference ranges across age groups in children enabling them to interact with more confidence with parents.
>
> Third, EWSs were seen as offering concrete evidence for professional concerns empowering nurses to overcome barriers to escalating care.
>
> Fourth, the EWS was seen as of little value in stable patients, those with baseline abnormal physiology and those experiencing neurologic deterioration.
>
> The authors conclude that: 'Combing an EWS with a clinician's judgement may result in a system better equipped to respond to deterioration than previous EWS studies focused on their test characteristics alone' (Bonafide et al., 2013, p. 252). Here then, research evidence points to the value of formalised processes and early warning algorithms used in conjunction with the professional judgements of clinicians.
>
> ---
>
> Bonafide, C.P., Roberts, K.E., Weirich, C.M., Paciotti, B., Tibbetts, K., Kerene, R. et al., 2013. Beyond statistical prediction: qualitative evaluation of the mechanisms by which pediatric early warning scores impact patient safety. J. Hosp. Med. 8(5), 248–253.

EXERCISE 8.10

> How do sensemaking processes impact on the project of interest and how is this distributed across participants? Here are some prompts to assist your thinking:
> What are the sensemaking mechanisms involved in the project work?
> When does sensemaking occur?
> What are the interpretative resources that are drawn upon?
> You can record your answer in the Care Trajectory Management Workbook (see Evolve website).

TABLE 8.1 ■ Core Components of the Translational Mobilisation Theory

Core Component	Definition	Subcomponent	Definition
Project	A sociomaterial network of collective action which follows a trajectory in time and space.	Primary project	The focus of collective action.
		Project actor	A defined social or material element within a project of action—technology, intervention, role.
Strategic action field	The context in which projects are progressed and which provide the social and material resources that condition collective action.	Structures	The stable elements of a strategic action field that generate the entities, positions and relationships through which an activity is organised (divisions of labour, hierarchies, departments, units, teams, interfaces).
		Organising logics	Elements of a strategic action field that provide a set of assumptions, values and beliefs that define the purpose and scope of possible action.
		Interpretative repertoires	The formal and informal meaning-making resources in the strategic action field: classifications, scripts, categories, mindlines, rules of thumb, pattern recognition, assessments.
		Materials	Elements of a strategic action field that provide the physical facilities, technologies and concrete resources to support an activity.
Mechanisms of mobilisation	Practices through which participants in a strategic action field progress projects.	Object formation	Practices through which objects of knowledge and practice are created and enrolled in collective action.
		Translation	Practices that allow different objects of practice and understandings to be shared to enable concerted action.
		Articulation	Practices that assemble and align the diverse elements (people, knowledge, materials, technologies, actions, bodies) through which projects are accomplished.
		Reflexive monitoring	Practices through which actors evaluate a field of action to generate awareness of project trajectories.
		Sensemaking	Practices though which actors interpret and create order in conditions of complexity and connect the fluidity of practice with organisational structures.

Developed from Allen, D., May, C., 2017. Organizing practice and practicing organization: towards an outline of translational mobilization theory. Sage Open. April–June 2017, 1–14. doi:10.1177/2158244017707993.

Summary

This chapter has described and explained the key components of TMT and their application to healthcare, using rescue trajectories as an illustrative case. TMT is a theory of emergent organisation that offers a way of seeing healthcare work that lays the foundations for understanding care trajectory management. It emphasises the agency of participants in systems of work, the fluidity of organisational processes, the sociomaterial distribution of activities and the reciprocal relationship between the everyday organisation of practice and the production of formal organisation. TMT provides a framework for thinking systematically about the networks of people, materials and technologies involved in a collective activity; the mechanisms of action through which activity is accomplished; and how action is shaped by the features of the strategic action field in which activity takes place. The core components of TMT are summarised in Table 8.1. The next chapter will build on this knowledge to illustrate how these theories and concepts can be used to explain and describe care trajectory management.

SUMMARY OF KEY LEARNING

- TMT is a theory and conceptual framework which describes and explains how collective activity is organised between people, materials and technologies, in unpredictable work environments.
- TMT is underpinned by the domain assumptions outlined in Chapter 7 and comprises three components: the project, the strategic action field and the mechanisms of mobilisation.
- The project is the unit of analysis in TMT; this defines the boundaries of the activity of interest for the purposes of the analysis.
- The concept of the strategic action field directs attention to the environments within which an activity takes place to consider how key contextual features (structures, materials, interpretive repertoires and organising logics) condition how the activity of interest is accomplished.
- In TMT the concept of mechanisms directs attention to how projects of collective action are mobilised and organised. These comprise of object formation, articulation, translation, reflexive monitoring and sensemaking.
- TMT provides a new way of seeing healthcare work and a framework for thinking systematically about the networks of people, materials and technologies involved in a collective activity, the mechanisms of action through which activity is accomplished and how action is shaped by the features of the strategic action field in which activity takes place.
- Combined with the ways of seeing healthcare outlined in TMT's domain assumptions (see Chapter 7), these theories and concepts can be used to intervene to bring about service improvements, and explain and describe care trajectory management.

QUICK QUIZ

- What is a project in TMT?
- What is a strategic action field in TMT?
- What are the four features of a strategic action field that impact on how an activity is accomplished?
- What are mechanisms of mobilisation in TMT?
- What is object formation?
- What is translation?
- What is articulation?
- What is reflexive monitoring?
- What is sensemaking?

References

Allen, D., 2016. The importance, challenges and prospects of taking work practices into account for healthcare quality improvement. J. Health Organ. Manag. 30 (4), 672–689.

Allen, D., Lloyd, A., Edwards, D., Grant, A., Hood, K., Huang, C., et al., 2022a. Development, implementation and evaluation of an early warning system improvement programme for children in hospital: the PUMA mixed-methods study. Health Soc. Care Deliv. Res. 10(1). doi:10.3310/CHCK4556.

Allen, D., Lloyd, A., Edwards, D., Hood, K., Chao, H., Hughes, J., et al., 2022b. Development, implementation and evaluation of an evidence-based paediatric early warning system improvement programme: the PUMA mixed methods study. BMC Health Serv. Res. 22 (1), 9.

Andrews, T., Waterman, H., 2005. Packaging: a grounded theory of how to report physiological deterioration effectively. J. Adv. Nurs. 52 (5), 473–481.

Bonafide, C.P., Roberts, K.E., Weirich, C.M., Paciotti, B., Tibbetts, K., Kerene, R., et al., 2013. Beyond statistical prediction: qualitative evaluation of the mechanisms by which pediatric early warning scores impact patient safety. J. Hosp. Med. 8 (5), 248–253.

Burke, J.R., Downey, C., Almoudaris, A.M., 2020. Failure to rescue deteriorating patients: a systematic review of root causes and improvement strategies. J. Patient Saf. 1 (18), e140–e155. doi:10.1097/PTS.0000000000000720.

Chua, W.L, Mackey, S., Ng, E.K.C., Liaw, S.Y., 2013. Front line nurses' experiences with deteriorating ward patients: a qualitative study. Int. Nurs. Rev. 60, 501–509.

Cioffi, J., 2000. Nurses' experiences of making decisions to call emergency assistance to their patients. J. Adv. Nurs. 32, 108–114. doi:10.1046/j.1365-2648.2000.01414.x.

Endacott, R., Westley, M., 2006. Managing patients at risk of deterioration in rural hospitals: a qualitative study. Aust. J. Rural Health. 14, 275–279. doi:10.1111/j.1440-1584.2006.00829.x.

Endsley, M.R., 1995. Toward a theory of situation awareness in dynamic systems. Hum. Factors J. 37 (1), 32–64.

Entwistle, V., 2004. Nursing shortages and patient safety problems in hospital care: is clinical monitoring by families part of the solution? Health Expect 7 (1), 1–5. doi:10.1046/j.1369-7625.2003.00259.x.

Fligstein, N., McAdam, D., 2011. Toward a general theory of strategic action fields. Sociol. Theory. 29, 1–26.

Gilson, R.D., 1995. Special issue preface. Hum. Factors. 37 (1), 3–4.

Goldenhar, L.M., Brady, P.W., Sutcliffe, K.M., Meurhing, S.E., 2013. Huddling for high reliability and situation awareness. BMJ Qual. Saf. 22 (11), 899–906.

Hernes, T., Maitlis, S. (Eds.), 2010. Process, Sensemaking and Organizing. Oxford University Press, Oxford.

Latimer, J., 2000. The Conduct of Care: Understanding Nursing Practice. Blackwell, Oxford.

Latour, B., 2005. Reassembling the Social: An Introduction to Actor-Network-Theory. Oxford University Press, Oxford.

Lydon, S., Byrne, D., Offiah, G., Gleeson, L., O'Connor, P., 2016. A mixed-methods investigation of health professionals' perceptions of a physiological track and trigger system. BMJ Qual. Saf. 25, 688–695. doi:10.1136/bmjqs-2015-004261.

Mackintosh, N., Sandall, J., 2010. Overcoming gendered and professional hierarchies in order to facilitate escalation of care in emergency situations: the role of standardised communication protocols. Soc. Sci. Med. 71 (9), 1683–1686.

Mackintosh, N., Watson, K., Rance, S., Sandall, J., 2014. Value of a modified early obstetric warning system (MEOWS) in managing maternal complications in the peripartum period: an ethnographic study. BMJ Qual. Saf. 23, 26–34. doi:10.1136/bmjqs-2012-001781.

May, C., Finch, T., 2009. Implementing, embedding and integration: an outline of normalization process theory. Sociology 43 (3), 535–554.

McDonnell, A., Tod, A., Bray, K., Bainbridge, D., Adsetts, D., Walters, S., 2013. A before and after study assessing the impact of a new model for recognizing and responding to early signs of deterioration in an acute hospital. J. Adv. Nurs. 69, 41–52. doi:10.1111/j.1365-2648.2012.05986.x.

Mol, A., 1999. Ontological politics: a word and some questions. In: Law, J., Hassard, J. (Eds.), Actor Network Theory and After. Blackwell Publishing, Oxford, pp. 74–89.

Mol, A., 2002. The Body Multiple: Ontology in Medical Practice. Duke University Press, Durham, NC.

Pattison, N., Eastham, E., 2012. Critical care outreach referrals: a mixed-method investigative study of outcomes and experiences. Nurs. Crit. Care. 17 (2), 71–82.

Roland, D., Oliver, A., Edwards, E.D., Mason, B.W., Powell, C.V.E., 2014. Use of paediatric early warning systems in Great Britain: has there been a change of practice in the last 7 years? Arch. Dis. Child. 99 (1), 26–29.

Sønning, K., Nyrud, C., Ravn, I.H., 2017. A survey of healthcare professional's experiences with the paediatric early warning score (PEWS). Norwegian J. Clin. Nurs. 12, e64605. doi:10.4220/Sykepleienf.2017.646 05en.

Strauss, A., Fagerhaugh, S., Suczet, B., Wiener, C., 1985. Social Organization of Medical Work. University of Chicago Press, Chicago, IL.

Weick, K.E., 1969. The Social Psychology of Organizing. Random House, London.

Weick, K.E., 1995. Sensemaking in Organizations. Sage Publications, London.

Suggested Reading

To find out more about TMT and its application to other areas of emergent organisation, see the website https://www.translationalmobilisationtheory.org.

Allen, D., 2018. Analysing healthcare coordination using translational mobilization theory. J Health Organ. Manag. 32 (3), 358–373.

This paper examines how TMT can be used for quality improvement purposes and has value on illustrating how care trajectory management knowledge can be deployed for advancing practice.

CHAPTER 9

Conceptualising Care Trajectory Management in Nursing Practice

LEARNING OUTCOMES

At the end of this chapter, you will be able to:
- Describe the three pillars of the care trajectory management framework
- Illustrate how the care trajectory management framework applies to nursing practice
- Explain the theoretical foundations of care trajectory management
- Use the care trajectory management framework to describe nursing practice

Introduction

Chapters 7 and 8 introduced Translational Mobilisation Theory (TMT) and a range of concepts and theoretical perspectives through which to understand, describe and explain the organisation of healthcare work. This chapter introduces the Care Trajectory Management (CTM) Framework, which builds on this thinking to provide a structure and language to explicate nursing's CTM function.

Development of the Care Trajectory Management Framework

The CTM Framework was developed by applying TMT in a secondary analysis of the data from *The Invisible Work of Nurses* (Allen, 2015) (Box 9.1). Taking CTM as the project of interest, I drew on TMT to conceptualise how patient care trajectories are managed and organised by nurses. While features of the *strategic action field* impact CTM, the primary purpose of the secondary analysis was to translate the tacit knowledge described in my original research into a conceptual framework that enabled this core nursing function to be more easily shared (Allen, 2019a, 2019b). Accordingly, the CTM Framework draws together the five TMT *mechanisms* to represent CTM processes and is designed to facilitate the formal integration of this critical nursing function into education and practice.

BOX 9.1 ■ Definition: Secondary Analysis

A secondary analysis entails examining existing data for purposes that differ from the original research. Secondary analysis is becoming more common in nursing research (O'Connor, 2020). For example, Leary et al.'s (2021) study of coroners' future prevention of death reports (see Chapter 5: Evidence From Future Prevention of Deaths Reports) was a secondary analysis of data produced for other purposes, and in the PUMA study (Allen et al., 2022a, 2022b) (see Chapter 8, Box 8.2), routinely collected hospital data were used to assess the impacts of the quality improvement intervention on patient outcomes.

PUMA, The Paediatric early warning system Utilisation and Morbidity Avoidance.

Allen, D., Lloyd, A., Edwards, D., Grant, A., Hood, K., Huang, C., et al., 2022a. Development, implementation and evaluation of an early warning system improvement programme for children in hospital: the PUMA mixed-methods study. Health Soc. Care Deliv. Res. 10(1). doi:10.3310/CHCK4556.

Allen, D., Lloyd, A. Edwards, D., Hood, K., Chao, H., Hughes, J. et al., 2022b. Development, implementation and evaluation of an evidence-based paediatric early warning system improvement programme: the PUMA mixed methods study. BMC Health Serv. Res. 22(1), 9.

Leary, A., Bushe, D., Oldman, C., Lawler, J., Punshon, G., 2021. A thematic analysis of the prevention of future deaths reports in healthcare from HM coroners in England and Wales 2016–2019. J. Patient Saf. Risk Manag. 26(1), 14–21. doi:10.1177/2516043521992651.

O'Connor, S., 2020. Secondary data analysis in nursing research: a contemporary discussion. Clin. Nurs. Res. 29(5), 279–284. doi:10.1177/1054773820927144.

BOX 9.2 ■ Care Trajectories and Care Trajectory Management

'Care trajectory' refers to 'the unfolding of a patient's health and social care needs, the total organisation of work carried out over its course, and the impact on those involved with that work and its organisation'. 'Care trajectory management' refers to the work of nurses in mobilising, coordinating and organising these relationships, to hold together and progress patient care.

The CTM Framework comprises three practice pillars:

Pillar 1: Trajectory awareness—practices involved in developing and maintaining an overview of trajectories of care as they evolve

Pillar 2: Trajectory working knowledge—practices involved in generating knowledge flows for CTM

Pillar 3: Trajectory articulation—practices involved in organising, aligning and mobilising care trajectory elements

The three pillars of CTM practice map on to TMT's mechanisms of mobilisation, summarised in Fig. 9.1.

The following section explores each of the three practice pillars in the CTM Framework. Scenarios from *The Invisible Work of Nurses* (Allen, 2015) will be used to illustrate the application of the framework to nursing practice. These examples are all drawn from the adult care context, as this was the location in which the original study was carried out. But the framework is relevant to all branches of nursing in the varied environments in which nurses work (Allen, 2019a). Before progressing any further, it might be helpful to refresh your understanding of care trajectories and CTM (Box 9.2).

The Three Pillars of Care Trajectory Management

PILLAR 1: TRAJECTORY AWARENESS

What Is Trajectory Awareness?

Trajectory awareness refers to the practices involved in maintaining oversight of trajectories of care as they evolve. It has parallels with the concept of situational awareness used in the safety

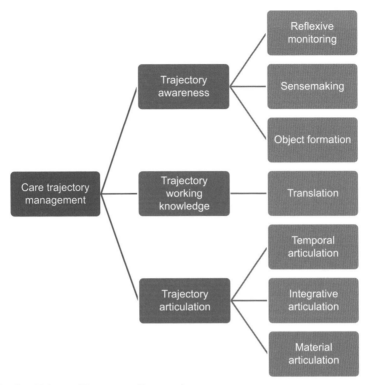

Fig. 9.1 The Care Trajectory Management Framework.

literature, which was considered in Chapter 8 in the discussion of rescue trajectories (see Box 8.5). But unlike the rescue trajectory example in which awareness relates to a discrete element of care (i.e., risk of deterioration), here we are concerned with how nurses develop an awareness of the whole patient trajectory. Trajectory awareness involves knowledge and understanding of an individual's health and care needs as well as any pertinent organisational issues. A senior nurse in *The Invisible Work of Nurses* (Allen, 2015) expressed this as 'knowing exactly what's going on everywhere'. This pithy description is very apposite, but arguably doesn't go far enough. Knowing exactly what is going on everywhere involves more than simply assembling a list of discrete actions and activities; it also includes understanding the sociomaterial relationships involved and their implications for practice.

Trajectory awareness is a fundamental prerequisite for CTM. Individual care trajectories evolve dynamically in response to changes in patients' health and social care needs, and shifts in the social, organisational and material arrangements associated with managing these needs. While some trajectories progress in a linear fashion in accordance with care and treatment plans, the dynamic interaction of the constituent elements can create unpredictability and knock trajectories off course. Winifred Naylor's recovery after hip fracture surgery was disrupted by the impact of a urinary tract infection (UTI) on her rehabilitation and delays in accessing community support services (see Chapter 2, Case Study 2.1); Edward Murphy's discharge planning was conditioned by the challenges of balancing Edward's needs and those of his wife, who was pregnant with twins (see Chapter 7, Case Study 7.1); and Gareth Williams's rehabilitation following a stoke was shaped by the effect of his injury on his mental health (see Chapter 3, Case Study 3.1). It is necessary to maintain awareness of trajectories as they evolve and intervene to modify arrangements as required. This can be challenging in a context in which facts and understanding pertinent to an

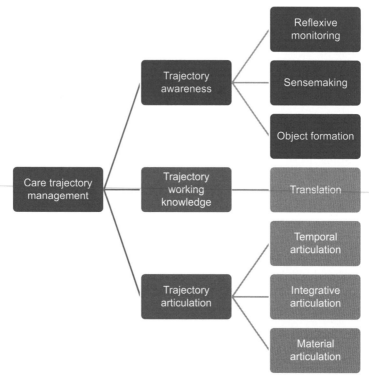

Fig. 9.2   Care Trajectory Management Framework pillar 1—trajectory awareness.

individual's care are distributed throughout the network of professionals, communities, artefacts and information technologies that comprise the healthcare system. It is also the case that nurses are typically responsible for managing multiple trajectories of care at any given time.

How Is Trajectory Awareness Achieved?

Maintaining trajectory awareness involves the TMT mechanisms of reflexive monitoring, sensemaking and object formation (Fig. 9.2).

Reflexive Monitoring. As described in Chapter 8 (see Reflexive Monitoring), reflexive monitoring denotes how the progress of a project of collective action is kept under review. In CTM this refers to the processes involved in maintaining oversight of an individual's care and treatment. This requires alertness and expertise in reading a complex field to recognise important clinical and organisational patterns and identify temporal and material constraints on action. It entails monitoring, noticing and assessing the salient aspects of individuals' care as these evolve and understanding when an intervention is indicated. It requires sensitivity to the organisational factors that are consequential for CTM, such as the arrangements which need to be in place for planned procedures, the materials that are required to support care and milestones that need to be achieved to facilitate progress. Beyond the patient, it involves attending to the status of the clinical environment and the activities of participants involved in the individual's care and assessing the implications for CTM. In addition to reflexive monitoring of the field, maintaining trajectory awareness involves drawing together information from a wide range of sources: formal documents, meetings, ward rounds or handovers, proactively solicited material and information generated

EXERCISE 9.1

Make a list of the sources of information that you would typically draw upon to understand a patient's evolving trajectory of care.

You can record your answer in the Care Trajectory Management Workbook (see Evolve website).

through interactions with patients, families and colleagues during everyday practice. Reflexive monitoring entails being attuned to and recognising the salience of these occasions. Before reading further, work through Exercise 9.1.

Sensemaking. Maintaining trajectory awareness also involves sensemaking (see Chapter 8: Sensemaking). In CTM this refers to the nursing activities involved in interpreting information pertinent to a trajectory (which may be clinical or organisational), identifying any inconsistencies, resolving gaps in understanding and detecting abnormal patterns and processes. Sensemaking, as Weick (1995) observes, may be triggered by a surprise, uncertainty or ambiguity. A record entry may not be clear, or an account of the case does not hang together, creates unease or provides an insufficient basis for action. Knowing where pertinent information is located, the trustworthiness of sources and the mechanisms of cross-validation is an important skill. Complete Exercises 9.2 and 9.3 to practise these skills.

There is considerable emphasis in nursing on the autonomous practitioner, but in everyday nursing work, sensemaking is regularly a collaborative activity. Collaborative sensemaking often draws on sources of knowledge and understanding which may not be formally documented in the patient record. This is illustrated in scenario 1 in Box 9.3, which is data from the silent handover study discussed in Chapter 6 (see Box 6.5) (Ihlebæk, 2020).

Beyond direct sources of information, in *The Invisible Work of Nurses* (Allen, 2015), nurses deployed pattern recognition, routines and standards to make sense of patient trajectories. Routines and standards have a contested place in professional practice and debates about their benefits and disbenefits turn on their role in mediating the relationship between the professional and the patient. For those who privilege evidence-based practice, standards are regarded as protecting patients against the idiosyncratic interventions of individual practitioners, such as those described by Bloor (1976) in his study on ear, nose and throat (ENT) surgeons (see Chapter 7, Box 7.6). For others, who prioritise patient centredness, standards are seen as generating cookbook practice and depersonalised care. These debates are a good reflection of the different organising logics that exist in healthcare systems. However, rather than allowing routines and standards to act as sites of tension in their application to a given case, we can more fruitfully focus on their value as resources in enabling nurses to make sense of practice. Trajectories that do not align with the patterns with which nurses are familiar can trigger the need for sensemaking. Standards and protocols are deployed and worked

EXERCISE 9.2

Review the list of information sources from Exercise 9.1 and rank them in terms of their trustworthiness.

You can record your answer in the Care Trajectory Management Workbook (see Evolve website).

EXERCISE 9.3

Review your answers to Exercise 9.2 and consider what strategies you would use to validate information from a source with uncertain credibility.

You can record your answer in the Care Trajectory Management Workbook (see Evolve website).

BOX 9.3 ■ Sensemaking in Action

Scenario 1: Collaborative Sensemaking

While the nurses sit at their computers, the conversation drifts into an oral report on particular patients (often referred to by room numbers). Nora says, 'You should pay extra attention to room 2. We didn't get to take her blood tests and provide her medication until rather late this morning, and she feels a bit neglected and frustrated'. 'Okay, I'll go and see her as soon as possible then', replies Eva and asks, 'Yesterday she seemed a bit feeble, even though her vitals were fine, how is she today?' Nora replies that she looks better and says she feels quite well. The results are satisfactory. Eva looks them up on the computer, making some notes on her paper patient list. 'Have you met her husband then?' Nora asks, raising her eyebrows. 'I know! A bit of a handful! I guess it's their way to get control though. We have to make sure to keep them both updated' Eva replies.

Ihlebæk (2020, p. 4)

Scenario 2: Routines and Sensemaking

SN1: I can't understand this transfer as she came in under Gynae, but she was under Urology. I didn't think you could transfer from an outlier to an outlier
SN2: You can't; not really!

(With permission from Allen, D., 2015. The Invisible Work of Nurses. Routledge, London and New York, p. 40.)

Ihlebæk, H.M., 2020. Lost in translation – silent reporting and electronic patient records in nursing handovers: an ethnographic study. Int. J. Nurs. Stud. 109. doi:10.1016/j.ijnurstu.2020.103636.

---

with flexibly as a reference point from which to make sense of a case for the purposes of progressing activity. In scenario 2 in Box 9.3, the staff nurse is scrutinising the patient record to make sense of a patient's trajectory. She is struggling to understand what has happened in this case as the history of the patient trajectory does not fit with her knowledge of organisational processes. In this sensemaking moment in the nurse's ordinary working day, we can see how her interpretative work could lead to a revised understanding of organisational processes, a deeper understanding of the circumstances of the case or both.

Some sensemaking activity is linked to formal occasions set aside for this purpose, such as making an entry into the patient record, participating in a team meeting or pausing to review the information displayed on a whiteboard. However, a large proportion of sensemaking is embedded in ongoing work processes, for which time is not formally allocated—such as corridor discussions, checking the availability of test results and through interaction with patients and their families. Although some caregiving tasks may not require a high degree of technical skill, they provide an opportunity for finding out and making sense of important information for the purposes of CTM, as well as other elements of patient care.

Object Formation. In maintaining trajectory awareness, the mechanisms of reflexive monitoring and sensemaking come together in object formation. In TMT, object formation refers to the mechanisms through which participants construct the focus of their practice to be able to do their work (see Chapter 8: Object Formation). For the purposes of direct patient care, nurses translate people into objects of nursing practice, through their nursing assessments. The review of activities of daily living and nursing risk assessments generates a singular construction of the patient as an object of nursing practice, the parameters of which are outlined in the care plan. For the purposes of CTM, however, object formation refers to the processes through which the *overall status of a care trajectory* is encapsulated, recorded and communicated to support its management. This extends beyond the understanding necessary to identify and attend to an individual's nursing care needs and includes information on the activities of other members of the healthcare team and the

EXERCISE 9.4

A Critical Reflection on 'Knowing the Patient'

Nurses often underline the importance of 'knowing the patient'. In formal theory this is taken to refer to the profession's distinctive biopsychosocial approach to patient care and reinforces ideas about emotional intimacy as the cornerstone of nursing practice (see Chapter 6, Box 6.2). The CTM Framework makes visible another dimension of holistic practice which includes *organisational* and *material* relationships as well as those developed with the patient and the family. Think about the content of the nursing admission and the information that is shared during nursing handover. What aspects of a patient's care and treatment are included? Is the content strictly limited to considerations of the patient's nursing care needs? What does this reveal about nursing's professional vision? When you use the term 'knowing the patient' in everyday practice, what exactly do you mean by this? What are the important aspects of the patient's care that you need to 'know'?

You can record your answer in the Care Trajectory Management Workbook (see Evolve website).

---

integration of clinical information about patient progress with organisational information necessary for the purposes of CTM.

This understanding is achieved through the creation of trajectory narratives, which encapsulate and summarise patients' overall ongoing care. When organisational actors are caught in the flow of time, narratives are a means of sustaining a coherent past (Hernes, 2014) and moving towards an agreed future. Trajectory narratives are typically started through the nursing admission process, consolidated through the nursing handover and adjusted contemporaneously in response to changes and developments in the person's care. Trajectory narratives have retrospective and prospective elements. They look back to summarise the history of the case and look forward to ongoing care and treatment.

Like sensemaking, maintaining trajectory narratives is often a collaborative activity in which nurses collectively review a patient, each adding elements to build up an overall picture. The personal notes made by nurses during handover and team meetings are in effect trajectory narrative 'plot summaries', which function as aide memoirs, and can be quickly updated as trajectories evolve.

Trajectory narratives are an important coordinating mechanism in healthcare systems; they generate an overview of a person's care, which incorporates the various sociomaterial elements and their relationships to produce an understanding of the whole which is greater than the sum of the individual parts. Such an understanding is essential for planning processes. There is no single place in the health and social care information and communication infrastructure where a trajectory summary is recorded, and no other healthcare professions take responsibility for maintaining this overall awareness. Before moving on to the next section, work through Exercise 9.4.

PILLAR 2: TRAJECTORY WORKING KNOWLEDGE

What Is Trajectory Working Knowledge?

Trajectory working knowledge refers to the role of nurses in creating the information flows and channels of communication that are necessary for the practical organisation of patient care trajectories. As a senior nurse in *The Invisible Work of Nurses* (Allen, 2015) described it: 'We're the link; they tell us and then we tell everyone else!'.

In the health informatics literature, a distinction is made between archival knowledge and working knowledge. *Archival knowledge* refers to information documented in the patient record which is typically oriented to the need to account for practice and is retained for future reference. *Working knowledge* is action oriented and generated to support the day-to-day organisation of the work (Fitzpatrick, 2004). The patient record is widely recognised as the primary mechanism of interprofessional communication in healthcare, and in recent years there has been significant investment in new information systems to support knowledge sharing, albeit with mixed results (Greenhalgh et al., 2019). Yet, while healthcare organisations tend to assume that the patient record can generate both archival and working knowledge, the information systems are designed primarily for the purposes of data recording and the requirements of clinical accountability, rather than to support the organisation of everyday work (see Chapter 3, Box 3.5). And this is where nurses fulfil an important coordinating role.

As explained in the previous chapter, when people enter healthcare systems, they are transformed into the objects of practice by the professions involved in their care (Chapter 8: Object Formation). Different professions have distinctive cognitive and practical concerns and make up patients in different ways. This produces the distributed, partial and fragmented understandings of the person that were described in Chapter 3 (see Complexity 3, Healthcare Is Distributed Work), which are then entered into the formal record. Because nurses work closely with patients and regularly interact with the participants involved in their care and treatment, they have a central role in bringing together these different versions of the patient, and in so doing they create the working knowledge that is required for CTM. Working knowledge refers to the shared understanding of patient trajectories that are produced for the purposes of practical action. Such agreements have different degrees of stability; some may have a high level of permanence and travel across time and space; other understandings might be relatively short-lived and confined to the requirements of a particular situation or decision-making context.

How Is Trajectory Working Knowledge Achieved?

Translation. Translation is the central mechanism involved in creating trajectory working knowledge (Fig. 9.3). In TMT 'translation' refers to the practices that enable differing viewpoints

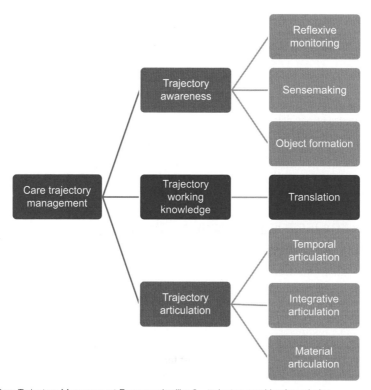

Fig. 9.3   Care Trajectory Management Framework pillar 2—trajectory working knowledge.

and multiple interests to be accommodated for activity to progress (see Chapter 8: Translation). While 'good' communication in health and social care is typically conceptualised in terms of the comprehensiveness of information, in practice successful trajectory management depends less on the exhaustiveness of information and more on ensuring that the right information is shared with the right people, in the right format, and that there is sufficient consensus between participants about the matters at hand to allow a trajectory to progress (Allen, 2015).

Translation depends on understanding the needs of organisational members so that information is presented in a form that is relevant and understandable. As described in the discussion of rescue trajectories in Chapter 8 (see Box 8.4), artefacts have an important purpose in supporting translational processes and can function to mediate communication between actors who do not have a shared language. One of the advantages of nurses' use of trajectory narratives in supporting information flows is that they can be modified for different audiences. *The Invisible Work of Nurses* (Allen, 2015) showed that nurses draw on their knowledge of the information requirements of team members to select relevant elements of the patient story. This is known as 'recipient design', which means that the information is tailored to the needs of the recipient. These skills are largely taken for granted in expert practice, but this sensitivity to the recipient design of narratives is revealed in scenario 1 in Box 9.4 by the nurse's 'repair'—'but you probably don't need to know that!'—which acknowledges that she has offered extraneous information to the doctor about the patient's dietary requirements when asked about this patient in the context of a ward round (see Box 9.4).

Translation depends on taking the perspective of others and understanding their information requirements. In psychology there is considerable evidence that people find perspective taking difficult (Heath and Staudenmayer, 2000). This challenge is particularly exacting in organisations where teams are ephemeral and staff cannot depend on prior relationships to facilitate understanding, or in circumstances in which the working worlds of actors are poorly understood or when communication is not face to face but mediated through alternative formats (e.g., telephone, written). This is important to understand, when one acknowledges that a major translational task for which nurses are largely responsible is the management of information across departmental and organisational boundaries to support transfers of care, where the nurse making the transfer may have only a fleeting acquaintance with the information requirements of the receiving service. In scenario 2 (see Box 9.4), the discharge

---

BOX 9.4 ■ Translation

Scenario 1: Perspective Taking and Recipient Design

Dr: and this new gent?
SN: [checks list] He has low BP and sore groins
Dr: Are we applying Canesten?
SN: its like a raised rash [reading from list] He's allergic to gluten, but you probably don't need to know that!
  (With permission from Allen, D., 2019b. Institutionalising emergent organisation in health and
    social care. Journal of Health Organization and Management. 33 (7/8), 764–775.)

Scenario 2: Translation Across Organisational Interfaces

Discharge Liaison Nurse locates a set of notes and flicks through a unified assessment form which has been completed. […] She complains that the information provided is insufficient and more details are required. In one section it simply states that a patient is incontinent of urine and faeces. Discharge Liaison Nurse says that this needs to include information on how this is managed. […] She said that one of the challenges for her was that there was a lack of understanding at ward level of the information that was required. Having looked through the unified assessment form Discharge Liaison Nurse makes an entry into the patient's notes requesting that more information is included and asks the ward to bleep her if they wish so that she can go through this with them.
  (With permission from Taylor & Francis Group. Allen, D., 2015. The Invisible Work of Nurses:
    Hospitals, Organisation and Healthcare. Routledge, London and New York, p. 120.)

liaison nurse is reviewing the unified assessment form, the document that was used in the study site for making referrals to social care. In the UK social carers work in the community to provide support to people who need assistance with everyday activities of living. Making an adequate referral required that hospital-based nurses provided detailed information on the person's ongoing care needs, to enable the social worker to assess whether the referral was appropriate and make a care plan.

Managing transitions of care is a substantial component of the nursing role which has important implications for healthcare quality and safety. This topic will be considered in more detail in the final chapter.

PILLAR 3: TRAJECTORY ARTICULATION

What Is Trajectory Articulation?

Nurses run the place. […] That requires anticipating people's needs and constantly being two steps ahead (Senior Nurse).

Allen (2015)

Trajectory articulation is the third pillar of the CTM Framework. It refers to the nursing practices through which the actions, knowledge and resources required to progress a trajectory of care are brought together when they are needed. Articulation can be proactive, with activity undertaken as part of a planned process, or responsive, where action is required to address an emergent issue. In the complex system of health and social care, decisions must be taken about what should be done, by whom, when, where and with what materials. Because patient care is often uncertain, emergent and unpredictable, and health and social care work is distributed in time and space, alignment of all the relevant elements of a patient's care cannot be taken for granted. The more elements that are involved, the more challenging this becomes.

Because of their proximity to the patient and unique trajectory awareness, nurses have a central role in articulating patient care. This requires organisational knowledge and understanding of processes and procedures, clinical expertise to anticipate how a trajectory will progress and skills in interprofessional working. Articulation work often requires that nurses assign work for others, either directly or indirectly, through mechanisms such as referral processes, doctor's job's books or whiteboards. Deciding on the urgency of the issue and the most appropriate mechanism of task allocation requires sensitivity to the work of others, particularly if this involves crossing professional boundaries.

How Is Trajectory Articulation Achieved?

CTM entails three kinds of articulation work. These are considered separately here but are often combined in practice (Fig. 9.4).

Temporal Articulation. Healthcare systems are complex temporal orders (Zerubavel, 1979). Certain services are provided 24 hours a day, 365 days a year, but many others operate on a more restricted basis. Some departments may only function at certain times of the day on specific days of the week or operate with limited capacity outside of core hours. Individual services have varying internal processes—such as the scheduling of meetings or the organisation of key activities—and professions and occupations have different working hours and shift patterns.

Temporal articulation is necessary to ensure actions and events take place at the right time and in the right order. *Proactive temporal articulation* is oriented to future needs. Many aspects of patient care—an operation, a procedure, a meeting, discharge, day hospital attendance—must be planned for to ensure that arrangements are in place to enable care to proceed. This requires an understanding of how the temporal organisation of the relevant components of the

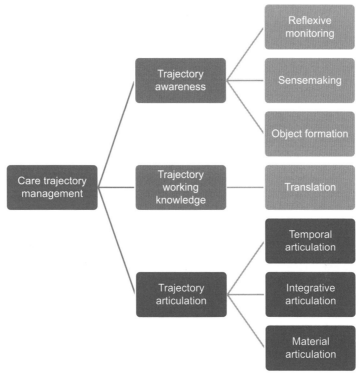

Fig. 9.4 Care Trajectory Management Framework pillar 3—articulation.

BOX 9.5 ▪ Proactive Temporal Articulation

Scenario 1

She said that in the afternoon she would look at the discharges planned for Thursday and see what needs to be done. 'So I can be proactively phoning the OT [occupational therapist] and the physio and getting them to come and do their assessments.

    (With permission from Taylor & Francis Group. Allen, D., 2015. The Invisible Work of Nurses: Hospitals, Organisation and Healthcare. Routledge, London and New York, p. 59.)

Scenario 2

Staff Nurse: 'I need to phone the GP (general practitioner/primary care doctor) about […].'
Coordinator: 'She's going home Monday isn't she?'
Staff Nurse: 'Yeah, but she's a Warfarin discharge.'

    (With permission from Taylor & Francis Group. Allen, D., 2015. The Invisible Work of Nurses: Hospitals, Organisation and Healthcare. Routledge, London and New York, p. 59.)

---

health and social care system will impact on organisational processes to ensure delays are not incurred. The examples in Box 9.5 are taken from *The Invisible Work of Nurses* (Allen, 2015). Scenario 1 is derived from my observations of a ward coordinator and shows the work involved in planning for discharge, and alerting other members of the team to any required actions. In scenario 2, which is derived from observations made at the nurses' station, the coordinator is puzzled by the actions of the staff nurse in contacting a primary care doctor for the purposes of discharge planning. In explaining her actions, the staff nurse indicates that this is not a routine

---

BOX 9.6 ■ Responsive Temporal Articulation

Scenario 1

Coordinator: 'Mr X, I think he's got a UTI. He was aggressive in the night. Do you want to start him on anything? [...] His temperature is 38.5, we can do cultures here [...].'
Junior Doctor: 'We could start him on Augmentin [antibiotic].'
Doctor writes the prescription.
 (With permission from Taylor & Francis Group. Allen, D., 2015. The Invisible Work of Nurses:
  Hospitals, Organisation and Healthcare. Routledge, London and New York, p. 60.)

Scenario 2

There is a note in the hospital at night book about a patient's blood sugar levels. The patient has been nil by mouth for 48 hours and is not on insulin but her blood glucose levels are increasing and she has ketones in her urine. The patient tells SNP the doctors have said they will not give her insulin until tomorrow. SNP checks the patient's notes and is not happy. She goes back to the patient and says she will ask the doctors to review her.
 (With permission from Taylor & Francis Group. Allen, D., 2015. The Invisible Work of Nurses:
  Hospitals, Organisation and Healthcare. Routledge, London and New York, p. 60.)

---

case; the patient is being discharged home on warfarin, and primary care requires advanced notice in such cases as they must plan for regular blood tests and medication management.

Whereas proactive temporal articulation is a necessary component of planned processes, *responsive temporal articulation* refers to the actions that are necessary to address unpredictable contingencies and events. The need for action might arise because of changes in the patient's condition, changes in the organisation or changes in the arrangements in an evolving trajectory of care. Because nurses maintain awareness of patient trajectories, other actors—particularly doctors—are dependent on them to be alerted to relevant issues.

In the first of the following examples (Box 9.6)—scenario 1—a ward nurse initiates a conversation with the junior doctor about commencing antibiotics on a patient with signs of a UTI. In scenario 2, a specialist nurse practitioner (SNP) from the Hospital at Night Team identifies the need for a medical review of a patient whose blood glucose levels are increasing.

Having identified the requirement for an intervention in the management of a trajectory, the urgency of the task must be assessed. These can be finely balanced decisions. Remember the case of Julie Carmen in Chapter 5 (Case Study 5.1) and the consequences for her recovery of not receiving antibiotics when these were required because the request fell through the gaps in the system.

Integrative Articulation. *Integrative articulation* is action undertaken to ensure decision making is joined up and individual trajectory elements cohere. When largely independent actors all contribute to patient care, decisions that seem reasonable in isolation can be problematic in the context of an overall trajectory of care. Writing in 1977 and observing increased specialisation in healthcare, Hockey (1977) observed: 'The nurse's contribution to care may lie, at least in part, in the promotion of a functional synthesis of disjointed endeavours' (p. 151, cited by Jackson et al., 2021). Reflecting on the work of nurses now and the impacts of coordination failures on healthcare quality, this has never been more important.

Because nurses maintain an overall trajectory awareness, they are attuned to the relationships between trajectory components and their interdependencies and have an important role in identifying and addressing these potential dangers. In our first illustration of this point (scenario 1, Box 9.7), the nurse contacts a doctor to clarify an earlier instruction to administer a dextrose infusion to a patient with diabetes. The nurse knows that the dextrose infusion was prescribed by the first doctor as a source of energy when it was assumed that the patient would be 'nil by mouth'. Now she is eating, it is no longer required, but the nurse has no authorisation to cancel

---

BOX 9.7 ■ Integrative Articulation

Scenario 1

Staff Nurse makes another call to another doctor to clarify earlier advice about a dextrose infusion and 2 hourly BMs [blood glucose monitoring] in the light of a decision taken by another team that the patient can eat and drink for now but will be nil by mouth from midnight.

(With permission from Taylor & Francis Group. Allen, D., 2015. The Invisible Work of Nurses: Hospitals, Organisation and Healthcare. Routledge, London and New York, pp. 68–69.)

Scenario 2

Junior doctor: 'We need to check the potassium I think and check the stool and then we can think about getting home. If I can sort out the paperwork you can go today if all's OK.' [The doctor makes as to leave the room and says almost as an afterthought]: 'How's the wound? I suppose I'd better check' [returns and examines the patient's abdomen].
Coordinator asks the patient: 'Have you done the stairs?'
Patient says he has.

(With permission from Taylor & Francis Group. Allen, D., 2015. The Invisible Work of Nurses: Hospitals, Organisation and Healthcare. Routledge, London and New York, p. 68.)

BOX 9.8 ■ Perceptions of Nurses' Attendance at Ward Rounds

A survey undertaken to inform the development of joint guidance on ward rounds undertaken in the UK by the Royal College of Physicians and Royal College of Nursing (RCN) found quite different perceptions of nurses' attendance on ward rounds (RCN, 2021): 9.3% of consultants on acute medical units and 17.7% on wards reported that the nurse looking after the patient was present on the ward round, with only 5.5% stating that this happened all the time. However, nurses across different units stated that they participated in ward rounds 61% of the time. Many also stated that they were so busy with patient care that it was impossible for them to join the ward round—despite wishing to do so. Nurses were sometimes perceived by medical staff to be too busy with nursing tasks for increasingly complex patients; however, nurses expressed frustration at not being always involved in wards rounds.

Critical Reflection: How might we account for the differences in the perspectives of consultants and nurses in the survey?

RCN, 2021. Modern Ward Rounds: Good Practice for Multidisciplinary Inpatient Review. RCN, London. https://www.rcn.org.uk/Professional-Development/publications/rcn-modern-ward-rounds-good-practice-for-multidisciplinary-inpatient-review-uk-pub009566 (Accessed 12 December 2023).

---

the doctors' request and the doctor has no way of knowing about the subsequent decision by the second medical team.

In scenario 2 (see Box 9.7), the nurse intervenes in discharge planning. In this example, the doctor informs the patient he can be discharged home. However, medical fitness is only one factor to be considered in reaching a discharge decision. The nurse is oriented to this and asks the patient whether they have had a mobility assessment: 'Have you done the stairs?' Although not directly questioning the doctor, her inquiry creates the opportunity for new information to be brought into the decision-making process.

Nurses' trajectory awareness and their role in supporting integrative articulation underline the importance of participation in planning meetings, whether this is hospital ward rounds, multidisciplinary team meetings or case conferences (Box 9.8). The evidence suggests that this can be challenging owing to competing clinical priorities, workforce gaps, organisational culture and skills, providing further evidence for the importance of formal recognition of nursing's CTM function.

Material Articulation. Healthcare work is distributed across people, technologies and artefacts (see Chapter 7: Domain Assumption 4: The Sociomaterial Distribution of Work). Material

---

BOX 9.9 ■ Material Articulation

Scenario 1

Staff Nurse: '[…] has gone down to 90 is there any chance you could go to 100 as they don't have 90 tablets and he's got to give them himself.'

Junior Doctor: 'When I increase it, it increases his epistaxis so it's likely to have to come down further.'

Staff Nurse: '80 – they do 80 tabs: OK so I can have a word with the registrar.'
    (Reproduced with permission from Taylor & Francis Group. Allen, D., 2015. The Invisible Work of Nurses: Hospitals, Organisation and Healthcare. Routledge, London and New York, p. 69.)

Scenario 2

Clinical Director: 'There's a man on [surgical ward] with hospital acquired pneumonia who we're going to have to connect. […] Which bed space do you want me to admit him to?'

Coordinator: 'He can go into [bed] 5. What drugs do you want?'

I missed the Clinical Director's response. Coordinator informed the nurse in the area and began checking the equipment, drawing up drugs and labelling them. […] Other nurses move into action, one covers the bed with paper sheets and a 'pac slide' [a device for moving patients], another is running through IV bags and connecting these to equipment. At one point five people are contributing to the preparations; each seems to know what they're doing and the division of labour occurs without any explicit discussion. […] Coordinator then checks the drugs she has drawn up with the nurse caring for the patient. Another nurse says: 'I have checked the trolley and its all fine'. [She was referring to the trolley with all the ventilator equipment on it].
    (Reproduced with permission from Taylor & Francis Group. Allen, D., 2015. The Invisible Work of Nurses: Hospitals, Organisation and Healthcare. Routledge, London and New York, p. 73.)

---

articulation refers to the practices required to ensure the availability, organisation and alignment of the physical resources involved in a trajectory of care. It includes the technologies and materials that support healthcare work, as well as the physical infrastructures and assistive technologies on which people depend for their everyday activities of living. Material articulation operates at several levels.

At one level, this mechanism is reflected in the role of nurses in maintaining oversight of the material arrangements that support patient care. In scenario 1 (Box 9.9), the nurse negotiates to modify a patient's medications as these do not come in tablet form in the dosage prescribed and the patient, who is about to be discharged home, is unable to break the tablets in half to administer the correct dose. This is a finely wrought judgement in which the nurse draws on her knowledge of the patient and the dose formats of this medication to identify the potential risks involved in discharging the patient home on his current prescription. Such interventions can be highly consequential for medication adherence and yet go largely unnoticed in the cacophony of decisions that shape trajectory management.

At another level, material articulation may involve aligning the arrangements for a particular procedure or activity. For acute time-critical events, this is evidenced in the use of artefacts such as resuscitation boxes, which ensure everything required in a medical emergency is available when it is needed. In this context, routine safety checks and maintaining stock levels are an important component of material articulation. While this may seem like a mundane activity, research on patient safety has repeatedly identified the unavailability of equipment or medications have contributed to catastrophic consequences (BBC, 2012; Telegraph Reporters, 2012). Many other areas of healthcare also depend on materials being assembled as required, and nurses make an important contribution to this work. Scenario 2 (see Box 9.9) is taken from observations in the intensive care unit, as the nursing staff swung into action to prepare the field for an admission.

Finally, material articulation requires attention to the context and infrastructure of care. In the community, this involves surveillance of the home environment to ensure patients have everything in place to support their care needs (Campling et al., 2022; Stokke et al., 2021). Seemingly mundane issues can throw homecare into disarray, and it is often community nurses who have an overview of the success or otherwise of continuing care arrangements (Melby et al., 2018; Norlyk et al., 2023). And while it might not be immediately obvious, bed management is an important and common example of material articulation. A 'bed' is not simply a physical artefact; it includes the associated expertise, materials, technology and infrastructures. Allocating patients to the most appropriate bed is one way of ensuring the availability of all the elements required to meet their care. Nurses are often employed in speciality bed management roles, but increasingly nurses across all areas of the healthcare system are being enrolled in the process of bed management, whether that is in allocating patients to beds in the acute sector, expediting a hospital admission or discharge or organising residential placements in the community. This involves skilful 'match-making' processes in allocating beds to meet patient needs. Chapter 10 considers in greater detail this aspect of nursing practice.

Care Trajectory Management in Action

In the previous section we have described and explained the three practice pillars of the CTM Framework. While the development of a framework is valuable for the purposes of describing and explaining CTM work, it is less good at conveying the gestalt, what it looks and *feels* like when all the different elements are brought together. This is because CTM is both a way of perceiving and reacting to the healthcare field as well as a set of knowledge-based practices. This chapter closes with an extended example (Case Study 9.1) of nursing's CTM in action. This is unpublished data from *The Invisible Work of Nurses* (Allen, 2015) study and is derived from observations of a community care coordinator (CCC). The role no longer exists within the organisation, but at the time, its purpose was to maintain an oversight of individuals with complex health conditions in the community, who had experienced recurrent health crises and were frequent contacts with the primary care doctors.

What began as a routine visit to monitor Cynthia's diabetes management evolved into a safety critical intervention in Cynthia's ongoing care. Beyond offering a very good illustration of the mechanisms of CTM in action, this example provides insight into the skills and knowledge of the CCC which underpin her CTM work. Her detection of the risks involved in the actions of the out-of-hours doctor was underpinned by not only a clinical understanding of trimethoprim but also her practical knowledge of the sociomaterial arrangements for Cynthia's ongoing care. Unlike the doctor, the care coordinator recognised the impossibility of removing the evening dose of trimethoprim from the blister packs. First, the trimethoprim cannot be safely distinguished from the other tablets Cynthia takes in the evening. Second, because of regulatory restrictions, carers are only allowed to prompt Cynthia to take her medication from the blister pack; they cannot not administer it. In addressing the risks in this scenario, the nurse's actions also demonstrate her knowledge of the key actors and agencies involved in this case: she contacts the care agency to obtain the code for the Dossett box so that this can be shared, and she attempts to contact the primary care doctor, so they can appraise the out-of-hours service of the situation. These are small interventions, with big consequences, and which display a sophisticated understanding of the network of relationships between the technologies, agencies and actors involved in Cynthia's trajectory of care (Exercise 9.5).

CASE STUDY 9.1 | Cynthia's Antibiotic Management

The first lady we are visiting today is 'Cynthia', an elderly woman who has diabetes and memory problems. The community care coordinator (CCC) explained that her diabetes is controlled with medication but that 'her blood sugars are all over the place'. The plan is to reduce the dose of diabetes medication. CCC has been asked to go in and 'monitor things'. She explains that Cynthia has carers to assist with washing and dressing and they are allowed to prompt her to take her medications, but they are not allowed to give them to her. Her medications are managed through blister packs. (Blister packs are a technology for helping people to keep track of their medications. Medications are dispensed weekly and combined in a designated sealed compartment or bubble to be taken at specific times of the day.)

We arrive at the flats where Cynthia lives and wait to be let in using the intercom system. On entry we are confronted by a wall of heat and CCC observes, 'crikey it's hot in here'. Cynthia is watching breakfast television and is still in her dressing gown. CCC asks how she is, and Cynthia says she is not well as she has a 'water infection' and is 'feeling a bit sick'. Cynthia says that she has contacted her primary care doctor who is coming to see her today, but that she has also been seen by 'another doctor' who prescribed her more tablets. She hands these to CCC; they are trimethoprim, an antibiotic used to treat urinary tract infections (UTIs). Someone has written on the medication box that these tablets are to replace the evening maintenance dose of the same drug Cynthia regularly takes, and which is included in her blister packs. CCC takes out a folder from the shelf under the television and reads through the notes. (This, I later found out, was the carers' folder.)

CCC: Here it says that on the 12th the doctor got them delivered but there's nothing here to say the trimethoprim was removed from the box. (The reference to 'box' in this utterance refers to a locked Dossett box, where Cynthia's medications are kept because of her memory problem, and which can only be accessed by the home carers.)

CCC is concerned and explains that there are several tablets to be administered at a given time and the carers are not able to remove the unwanted drug from the blister pack. Therefore, with the new prescription, the dose of trimethoprim Cynthia is receiving is too high, which could cause renal failure. In addition, because of Cynthia's memory problems, all medications should be kept in the locked Dossett box. CCC explained that part of the problem was that Cynthia was being seen by out-of-hours primary care doctors who 'had only part of the picture' and would not appreciate some of the challenges with her memory or the practical challenges involved in her medication management. CCC suggests to Cynthia that she stops taking the trimethoprim.

CCC then makes a call to the home care agency to obtain information on the code to access the Dossett box to enable this to be shared with the out-of-hours primary care doctors so they can change the contents of her medications if necessary. She explains the problem created by the prescription of trimethoprim by the out-of-hours doctor and confirms with the care agency that carers are not allowed to remove medications from the blister packs.

We return to the sitting room, and CCC then attempts to contact Cynthia's primary care doctor to discuss the issues with the out-of-hours team, but she learns that the doctor is seeing a patient. Initially, she says she will hold, but after a minute or so, she is informed that the doctor is likely to be 5 minutes or more and suggests that the doctor calls her back.

CCC then turns attention to taking Cynthia's blood glucose reading which is the purpose of the visit. She spends some time searching her bag for reagent sticks. As she is searching, Cynthia turns to me and says: 'Don't get old dear'.

EXERCISE 9.5

Reread Case Study 9.1 and use the CTM Framework to identify the TMT mechanisms of involved in this scenario. Imagine you are a qualitative researcher, analysing the data to locate evidence of the practice pillars and mobilisation mechanisms from the CTM Framework.

You can record your answer in the Care Trajectory Management Workbook (see Evolve website).

Summary

This chapter has introduced the CTM Framework, which provides a structure and language with which to articulate this safety critical element of nursing practice. Real-life data drawn from *The Invisible Work of Nurses* (Allen, 2015) have been used to illustrate the core components and mechanisms of

CTM work, including an extended integrated example centred on Cynthia's care (see Case Study 9.1). CTM is a complex process and always more than the sum of its parts. The final chapter synthesises this learning and considers its application in practice.

SUMMARY OF KEY LEARNING

- The care trajectory framework was developed by applying TMT to undertake a secondary analysis of the data from *The Invisible Work of Nurses* (Allen, 2015).
- The framework has three practice pillars: trajectory awareness, trajectory working knowledge and trajectory articulation.
- CTM is more than the sum of its parts.

QUICK QUIZ

- What is trajectory awareness?
- What are the three mechanisms involved in developing and maintaining trajectory awareness?
- What is trajectory working knowledge?
- What is the mechanism involved in developing trajectory work knowledge?
- What is trajectory articulation?
- What are the three forms of trajectory articulation?

References

Allen, D., 2015. The Invisible Work of Nurses. Routledge, London and New York.

Allen, D., 2019a. Care trajectory management: a conceptual framework for formalising emergent organisation in nursing practice. J. Nurs. Manag. 27 (1), 4–9.

Allen, D., 2019b. Institutionalising emergent organisation in health and social care. J. Health Organ. Manag. 33 (7/8), 764–775.

BBC., 2012. Secret Scottish NHS incident reports released. Retrieved from http://www.bbc.co.uk/news/uk-scotland-20395257 (Accessed 14 December 2022).

Bloor, M., 1976. Bishop Berkeley and the adenotonsillectomy enigma: an exploration of variation in the social construction of medical disposals. Sociology 10 (1), 43–61.

Campling, N., Birstwistle, J., Richardson, A., Bennett, M.J., Meads, D., Santer, M., et al., 2022. Access to palliative care medicines in the community: an evaluation of practice and costs using case studies of service models in England. Int. J. Nurs. Stud. 132, 104275.

Fitzpatrick, G., 2004. Integrated care and the working record. Health Inform. J. 10, 291.

Greenhalgh, T., Wherton, J., Shaw, S., Papoutsi, C., Vijayaraghavan, S., Stones, R., 2019. Infrastructure revisited: an ethnographic case study of how health information infrastructure shapes and constrains technological innovation. J. Med. Internet Res. 21 (12), e16093. doi:10.2196/16093.

Heath, C., Staudenmayer, N., 2000. Coordination neglect: how lay theories of organizing complicate coordination in organizations. Res. Organ. Behav. 22, 155–193.

Hernes, T., 2014. A Process Theory of Organization. Oxford University Press, Oxford.

Hockey, E., 1977. The nurses' contribution to care in a changing setting. J. Adv. Nurs. 2 (2), 147–156.

Ihlebæk, H.M., 2020. Lost in translation – silent reporting and electronic patient records in nursing handovers: an ethnographic study. Int. J. Nurs. Stud. 109. doi:10.1016/j.ijnurstu.2020.103636.

Jackson, J., Anderson, JE., Maben, J., 2021. What is nursing work? A meta-narrative review and integrated framework. Int. J. Nurs. Stud. 122, 103944. doi:10.1016/j.ijnurstu.2021.103944.

Melby, L., Obstfelder, A., Hellesø, R., 2018. 'We tie up the loose ends': homecare nursing in a changing healthcare landscape. Glob. Qual. Nurs. Res. 5. doi:10.1177/2333393618816780.

Norlyk, A., Burau, V., Ledderer, L.K., Martinsen, B., 2023. Who cares? The unrecognised contribution of homecare nurses to care trajectories. Scand. J. Caring Sci. 37, 282–290.

Stokke, R., Melby, L., Isaksen, J., Obstfelder, A., Andreassen, H., 2021. A qualitative study of what care workers do to provide patient safety at home through telecare. BMC Health Serv. Res. 21 (1), 553. doi:10.1186/s12913-021-06556-4.

Telegraph Reporters, 2012. Patients die due to flat batteries in hospital equipment. Retrieved from http://
    https://www.telegraph.co.uk/news/health/news/9589157/Patients-die-due-to-flat-batteries-in-
    hospital-equipment.html (Accessed 8 December 2022).
Weick, KE., 1995. Sensemaking in Organizations. Sage Publications, London.
Zerubavel, E., 1979. Patterns of Time in Hospital Life. Chicago University Press, Chicago, IL.

Suggested Reading

The Application of TMT to CTM

Allen, D., 2018. Translational Mobilisation Theory: a new paradigm for understanding the organisational elements of nursing work. Int. J. Nurs. Stud. 79, 36–42.

This paper shows how TMT can be used to understand the organisational aspects of nursing practice. This was a prerequisite for the development of the CTM Framework.

Allen, D., 2018. Care Trajectory Management: a conceptual framework for formalising emergent organisation in nursing practice. J. Nurs. Manag. 1, 4–9. doi:10.1111/jonm.12645.

This article builds on the TMT paper to offer a succinct framework for communicating and explaining the organisational components of nursing work. Here, the concept of CTM is deployed for the first time to conceptualise the organisational component of nursing work which has previously had no name.

CHAPTER 10

Care Trajectory Management in Nursing Practice

LEARNING OUTCOMES

At the end of this chapter, you will be able to:

- Describe the competencies that underpin care trajectory management
- Apply the Care Trajectory Management Framework to make sense of and plan activity in a clinical case load
- Understand the nursing contribution to care transitions
- Understand the nursing contribution to the organisation of infrastructures of care
- Understand the nursing contribution to trajectory stabilisation
- Assess patient care trajectories
- Use the language of care trajectory management to discuss nursing practice and lead a service improvement process
- Understand the opportunities for advancing practice and improving services
- Assess personal care trajectory management competence and identify continuing professional development needs

Introduction

The last nine chapters have covered a wide terrain to examine the centrality of care trajectory management (CTM) in the nursing role, its importance for the quality and safety of patient care and the reasons for, and the consequences of, its invisibility in nursing practice. Translational Mobilisation Theory (TMT) and the CTM Framework provide conceptual resources with which to describe and explain the complexity and organisation of healthcare work and the mechanisms involved in managing trajectories of care. This closing chapter consolidates this learning, by considering the application of these ideas to practice, professional development planning and advancing the nursing contribution to healthcare systems.

Care Trajectory Management Competencies

This section reviews the competencies that underpin CTM. While these have been implicit in earlier discussions, it is nursing practices that have been our primary focus to date. Here, we shift attention to the *practitioner* and the skills and competencies underpinning this core nursing function. Some CTM competencies are generic and inform the totality of CTM, and some are specific and relate to the individual pillars of the CTM Framework. This section draws on a previously published paper which explored strategies for integrating preparation for CTM into nurse education (Allen et al., 2019).

GENERIC CARE TRAJECTORY MANAGEMENT COMPETENCIES

This section examines the generic competencies that are required for all aspects of CTM work.

Theoretical and Conceptual Competence

A core theme of this book has been the importance of theories and concepts to describe and reflect on nursing practice. As outlined in Chapter 1 (see Making the Invisible, Visible: Why Concepts Matter for Nursing Practice), the ability to see is not just a property of the eye or brain but is linked to discursive practices and classificatory systems (Goodwin, 1994). Developing competence in TMT and the CTM Framework provides a language and concepts to explain nursing work, describe trajectories of care and explicate the actions undertaken in support of high-quality care for patients and families. Theoretical and conceptual competence is also a prerequisite for helping learners see what experienced practitioners can see, and for enabling nurses to contribute to service improvement initiatives based on the work as it is done.

Interleaving Clinical, Organisational and Care Trajectory Management Competence

While CTM is the primary focus of this text, throughout, I have emphasised that CTM must be understood as interleaved with direct patient care and the work involved in maintaining the clinical environment or caseload. This interleaving entails a distinctive professional 'habitus' (Bourdieu, 1980). It requires the ability to zoom in and attend to individual patients, zoom out to review the wider clinical context and combine this knowledge in the management of care. Zooming in involves developing and maintaining a full clinical picture of all patients in the nurse's caseload and identifying the practical, social and concrete activities that must be organised to meet patient needs. Zooming out involves maintaining an awareness of any constraints on this activity—the temporal organisation of services, the sequencing of actions, shifting patterns of demand in the clinical environment, accessibility of personnel, regulatory frameworks and the availability of equipment—and building these considerations into trajectory planning.

Health and Social Care Systems Competence

Knowledge of health and social care systems is a further prerequisite for CTM. This requires the capacity to look beyond patients' immediate nursing needs to consider their wider network of care and understand its implications for CTM. This includes developing an understanding of patients' social arrangements and informal sources of support. It also involves identifying the organisations and services involved, and understanding the legislative, policy and regulative frameworks within which they operate and their implications for the organisation of care. Health and social care systems expertise develops over time with progressive familiarity with a clinical service and the population served. While local intelligence of this kind is highly valued, it is also quickly disrupted when nurses move to new practice areas (Allen, 2015). Systems competence does not necessarily entail an encyclopaedic knowledge of a health and social care ecology but the capacity to adopt a systems perspective and the skills to locate and assess this information as it is required.

Relational Competence

CTM is inherently relational. The importance of relationships with patients and families is emphasised in clinical practice, but CTM depends too on managing relationships with a wide range of organisational actors. This includes the ability to interact and communicate across professional boundaries and organisational hierarchies, and skills in mediating different interests and perspectives (Allen, 2004). Relational competence also demands an understanding of the roles and responsibilities of healthcare providers, the knowledge and confidence to act as an equal partner in the team and highly developed communication skills in taking the perspective of others and translating information into content that is tailored to the situation and recipient.

Complexity Management Competence

Whether in the acute hospital, the community, care home or another setting, successful CTM requires nurses to be able to function in conditions of uncertainty. This involves an understanding of planned and emergent forms of organisation (see Chapter 4) and the ability to recognise when routines, standards and protocols are appropriate mechanisms for organising care and when bespoke approaches and professional judgements are called for. Functioning in complex circumstances also depends on having the skills to manage a caseload, to balance the needs of individuals with the needs of whole populations and to demonstrate a critical sensitivity to the ethical dimensions and consequences of prioritising care. The ability to make a cognitive and psychological shift from the high levels of alertness and vigilance necessary to maintain trajectory awareness to being present in the moment for patients and families in attending to their needs is essential. Tolerance of unpredictability, the ability to work flexibly, resourcefulness, problem solving and agility in responding to contingencies and evolving care needs are additional vital competencies in this context.

Information and Communications Competence

Expertise in working with information and communications systems is another essential skill. CTM depends on the ability to navigate information infrastructures and proficiency in the use of a range of paper-based and digital technologies to access, input and share information within teams and between agencies. Healthcare and social care are knowledge-intensive systems of work. The absence of information and communications capability is as consequential for the quality and safety of patient care as the absence of clinical skills. Information infrastructures evolve and there are likely differences between organisations and settings. Therefore, maintaining information, communication and digital skills is as important as updating clinical skills and should be reflected in nurses' continuing professional development strategies.

PILLAR-SPECIFIC CARE TRAJECTORY MANAGEMENT COMPETENCIES

Maintaining Trajectory Awareness Competence

Maintaining trajectory awareness requires the ability to identify the social, material and organisational elements that comprise individual trajectories of care, understand their interrelationships and be able to encapsulate this for the purposes of CTM. This includes skills in trajectory assessment and the capacity to recognise sources of actual or potential trajectory complexity, and to build this understanding into work planning and trajectory management.

Reflexive monitoring and sensemaking are central components of maintaining trajectory awareness and depend on the nurse's capacity to recognise clinical and organisational indicators that are consequential for CTM. At the level of the patient, this entails monitoring, noticing and assessing salient aspects of care as these evolve and identifying when action is required. At the level of the organisation or care environment, it entails alertness to the impact of shifting patterns of demand and organisational capacity on CTM, surveillance of the fit between infrastructural arrangements and patient care needs and identification of any constraints on action. Reflexive monitoring and sensemaking at both levels depend on the aptitude to proactively identify, access, interpret and synthesise relevant information; identify any gaps in understanding; and address any discrepancies. They depend too on alertness and expertise in reading a complex field to identify important clinical and organisational indicators that have implications for action.

Creating Working Knowledge Competence

Creating working knowledge depends on communication and relational skills so pertinent information is shared in an appropriate format, across lay, professional and service boundaries. It includes the activities involved in supporting everyday information flows between the range of actors interacting around the patient and the work of managing transfers of care. Both require an appreciation of the different understandings of a patient that comprise a trajectory; the ability to encapsulate this into a trajectory narrative; translational skills in interacting across professional, departmental and organisational interfaces; and competence in communicating information to enable the receiving party to do their work. In the case of everyday information flows, it additionally requires skills in prioritising action, recognising those elements of a trajectory that need to be shared to facilitate the organisation of the work, as well as an awareness of the wider demands and commitments of participants. In the case of patient transfers or transitions, it demands an understanding of how individual needs are mediated by the new environment of care. An overall essential competency in this context is relational knowledge of roles and responsibilities and the skills of perspective-taking to understand the information needs and work purposes of others. Highly developed oral, written and digital communication competencies—including an understanding of the strengths and limitations of different media—are essential.

Trajectory Articulation Competence

Competence in maintaining trajectory awareness and creating working knowledge are prerequisites for trajectory articulation. Additional specific competencies underpin different kinds of articulation work.

Temporal articulation requires an understanding of the work of professions, departments and units involved in a trajectory and their time-based organisation. It also depends on skills in identifying relevant organisational routines and procedures and assessing their implications for trajectory management. Routines and standards are a valuable sensemaking resource in complex and turbulent environments, which release cognitive capacity to address the nonstandard trajectories. Understanding the value of standards and protocols in each trajectory and recognising when these are a poor fit with the needs of patients and having the ability to explain such decisions are important skills. In some circumstances routines will be very familiar, but in others not; a reflexive awareness of such knowledge gaps and how to address this is also essential.

Integrative articulation is founded on the capacity to assess a care trajectory holistically to recognise possible contradictory or conflicting decisions, communicate this to the relevant party and reach a resolution. This demands comprehension of complex clinical presentations and organisational arrangements and the skills and confidence to raise and elucidate pertinent issues with the relevant parties.

Material articulation requires the ability to identify and locate the relevant resources necessary for addressing patient needs (materials, technologies, physical infrastructure, knowledge and expertise) and understand their interrelationships and implications for CTM. Material arrangements are often routinised and standardised; awareness of these plug-and-play arrangements is an important skill particularly in time-critical situations.

This is a long list of competencies, which must be brought together in CTM (see Table 10.1). These skills take time to develop; the aim of stipulating them here is to support continuous professional development planning. A self-assessment template is available in the Care Trajectory Management Workbook (Care Trajectory Management Competencies Professional Development Assessment Framework) (see Evolve website).

TABLE 10.1 ■ Care Trajectory Management Competencies

Level	Competency	Practices
Generic care trajectory management competencies	Theoretical/conceptual competence	• Understand Translational Mobilisation Theory. • Apply Translational Mobilisation Theory to healthcare organisation. • Understand the care trajectory management framework. • Apply the care trajectory management framework to practice.
	Interleaving clinical and organisational work competence	• Develop and maintain a full clinical picture of patients assigned to care. • Identify the practical, social and concrete activities necessary for meeting identified patient needs. • Develop a plan for the organisation of care considering potential system constraints.
	Health and social care systems competence	• Look beyond the patient and their immediate nursing needs to understand their wider formal and informal network of care and the professions, agencies and organisations involved and their implications for care trajectory management. • Understand the legislative, policy and regulative frameworks within which trajectory actors operate.
	Relational competence	• Understand the perspectives of those involved in a patient's care. • Understand the roles and responsibilities of the health and social care teams. • Interact and communicate across professional and organisational boundaries and hierarchies. • Mediate the relationships and interests involved in organising care around the wishes and needs of patients and families. • Translate information and tailor communications to meet the needs of the recipient.
	Complexity management competence	• Work in conditions of uncertainty and turbulence. • Understand planned and emergent forms of organisation. • Identify when routines and guidelines should be applied and where more responsive and bespoke approaches are indicated. • Manage patient caseload and prioritise care. • Make cognitive and psychological shifts from high levels of alertness and vigilance and being present in the moment for patients and families. • Flexibility, resourcefulness, problem solving and being able to respond to shifting demand patterns.
	Information and communications competence	• Competence in the use of paper-based and digital technologies. • Competence in navigating unfamiliar ICT systems.
Function specific care trajectory management competencies	Trajectory awareness competence	• Identify the social, material and organisational arrangements comprising a patient's care. • Encapsulate and summarise patient trajectories for different audiences. • Identify potential sources of trajectory complexity and build this into care planning. • Reflexive monitoring of patient's evolving care and organisation and understanding the implications of these relationships. • Making sense of complex information sources, identifying gaps and/or inconsistencies and implementing strategies for resolving these.
	Creating working knowledge competence	• Perspective-taking and the utilisation of relational and communication skills to mobilise the right information in the right format for the appropriate audience in a timely fashion.

Continued

TABLE 10.1 ■ Care Trajectory Management Competencies—cont'd

Level	Competency	Practices
	Trajectory articulation competence	• Understand the work of others involved in a trajectory of care. • Identify and appropriately use organisational routines to make sense of and articulate care trajectories. • Holistic assessment of patient trajectories and the comprehension of clinical and organisational relationships. • Identify the material arrangements necessary to support patient needs. • Bed management.

ICT, information communication technology.

Developed from Allen, D., Purkis, M.E., Rafferty, A.M., Obstfelder, A., 2019. Integrating preparation for care trajectory management into nurse education: competencies and pedagogical strategies. Nurs. Inq. 26(3), e12289. doi:10.1111/nin.12289.

Care Trajectory Management in Nursing Practice

This section focuses on CTM in nursing practice. It begins with the application of the CTM Framework to managing a caseload, before moving on to consider in detail some core CTM activities (managing transitions, optimising infrastructures of care, assessing trajectory complexity and 'talking CTM'). Each subsection has companion exercises, all of which are based on Transcript 10.1. This is a transcript of a nursing handover derived from previously unpublished data generated

TRANSCRIPT 10.1

Staff Nurse 1: Bed 1, Mark Haven, forty-five, came in with chest pain. Query pericarditis. He had an echo – there was nothing on it. What else has he had? Erh mmm – a VQ scan – nothing on that either. Nothing at all. He's complaining of a lot of pain. He's been written up for painkillers [...] and he can have it IM or IV. They'd rather he had it IM. He's also on Salbutamol nebulisers. No further plans. They've said when the pain has settled, he can go home.

Staff Nurse 1: Bed 2, Sebastian Turner. Eighty-four. He's really vague. We're not doing anything. He had a CT scan and that showed lots of haematoma and blobby bits. They thought he had a brain tumour. They've referred him to Robinson Ward for mobilisation and rehab, they should have a bed today. Sorry I didn't get around to sorting out the paperwork. I asked him what he'd had for breakfast this morning and he said: 'I used to be a mathematician twenty years ago and now I can't even remember what I had for breakfast'!

Staff Nurse 2: What is his home situation?

Staff Nurse 1: (scrutinises notes) He lives at home with a package of social care, family live locally but have raised concerns about whether he can cope. There's a contact number for the social worker.

Staff Nurse 1: Bed 3, Kevin Potter, seventy-six. On BGs – he was not known to be a diabetic until he came in. He came from a nursing home, and he has osteomyelitis. He hasn't got much idea about his diet, and I don't think he wants to either. 'Oh I'd like a lovely piece of cake'!. He has a chronic wound on his leg, which needs redressing. He's got an appointment this afternoon at the wound clinic which was arranged before he came in.

Staff Nurse 2: What time?

Staff Nurse 1: 1430.

Staff Nurse 1: In the next bed is Martin Blackmore, thirty-five. He has a right hemiplegia. He has a past medical history of a cerebral cyst in 1984. He's for a CT scan today. If it's to be something bad the wife and the son don't want them to go straight in and tell him. They want to be there.

Staff Nurse 2: Does he need to be nil by mouth for the scan?

Staff Nurse 1: I'm not sure to be honest. It's not until 2 o'clock.

Staff Nurse 1: Bed 5 is Brian Lowes, eighty-seven. The doctors have said that he can go. He's a lot better – up and walking to the toilet and less confused than he was but whether he's OK to go home I don't know. He's having an OT dressing assessment tomorrow. I don't know whether the physio has done a stairs assessment. Daughter says that if he can't pass the stairs assessment, they can bring the bed downstairs, but will need advance notice. He already had carers going in twice a day, but that might need increasing.

Staff Nurse 2: Do we have a planned discharge date?

Staff Nurse 1: It says Thursday here, but whether that is realistic?

Staff Nurse 1: Next is Jackson Mitre – a lovely sixty-two-year-old who came in with ascites that he's had for the past two months. He was discharged home two weeks ago but things have gone downhill again. He has shortness of breath, he's deaf and wears a hearing aid. He's got an artificial foot which he's had since he was two. He's a known epileptic. There are no real plans. He's for a chest X-ray today and has been referred to the neurology team. That's my lot.

Staff Nurse 3: Bed 7 is Norman Hollingsworth, sixty-two. He came in with diarrhoea and a low blood pressure. He's been on IV antibiotics over the weekend. (Reading from the notes) No diarrhoea for two days and his BP is 130/90. Now what else is there with him? Nothing really – he says that he feels like a new man today.

Staff Nurse 3: Bed 8, Hamish Drew, eighty-six with an old CVA. He came in with a chest infection. He's on an IVI. He can have a pureed diet and thickened fluids or normal fluids on a teaspoon. We're planning for home with him. He has a catheter which he is by-passing.

Staff Nurse 3: Next is Carlton Regis known as 'Tony'. Sixty-two. Came in following a collapse. He had a funny turn this morning. He dropped his BP and had an irregular pulse. Seen by the doctor, who is not overly concerned, thinks its most likely paroxysmal atrial fibrillation. He's started on a twenty-four-hour tape, and we need to start a twenty-four-hour urine when we get some acid. He's very anxious and his son has put in a formal complaint about the medical – not the nursing – staff because nothing was done over the weekend.

Staff Nurse 4: OK. I'll look out for them today.

Staff Nurse 3: Bed 10, Mohammad Kaif, sixty-three. He is an old MI who came from the cardiac ward. He's had one episode of chest pain this morning which was relieved by GTN. He does not speak any English but he has a word board and his family are in a lot.

Staff Nurse 4: Do his family do a lot for him?

Staff Nurse 3: Well he's pretty independent with his care. He can attend to his own hygiene needs. The word board is very good and he uses that. They add words to it as well – like pain. So that's growing.

Staff Nurse 3: Bed 11, Ian Howells, fifty eight. Came in with acute shortness of breath and chest pain. He's definitely had a PE. He's started on Warfarin and is for an exercise tolerance test and then he can go home. He will need TTHs writing up.

Staff Nurse 3: Bed 12, Edward Logan, ninety-two. Came in with reduced mobility and constipation. He's not constipated any more. He was seen by the social worker. His wife can't cope with him, and he's also told the social worker that he can't cope and yet he's done all his hygiene needs this morning. He wants to go into a care home. I've written my nursing assessment and the doctors have got to do their assessment.

Staff Nurse 3: Bed 13, David Lister, sixty-seven. Came in with increased shortness of breath. He's a known COPD. He's not very well. They've increased his nebulisers to six times a day. Doctor has asked to meet with his wife to discuss palliative care options. He's DNAR.

Staff Nurse 3: Bed 14 Donald Evans – 94. End stage COPD. He's DNAR now – as of yesterday. He told the doctors he wanted to die. The nephew is looking for a nursing home – Polar View, but there are four before him on the (waiting) list.

Continued

TRANSCRIPT 10.1—cont'd

Staff Nurse 4: He's getting depressed and needs to be nearer to home for people to visit. So I think we should think about referring him to Foxton Community Hospital. Otherwise, he is going to die here which is not appropriate.

Staff Nurse 3: Bed 15, Lionel Black. Going home today. TTHs dispensed. Nina could not book an ambulance yesterday as she was trying to get hold of the social workers to find out when the care package started. She called back at 5! So can we book an ambulance for 1 pm. His wife knows. All we need to do is to confirm with the dietician to see if she has done the referral for going home with thickener. We also need to send thickener with him as well. Oh, one more thing. During handover, his wife showed us fresh blood coming from his cough. It was in a tissue. He saw the doctor who was not concerned and thought it had just come from coughing.

Staff Nurse 3: Bed 16 — Hugh Thomas   86   admitted with a chest infection and came to us from Bluebell Ward. They apparently said he was mobilising independently but with us when he mobilised to the toilet he was very unsteady and yesterday was very drowsy. So not sure what's going on there. We are just waiting for a (cognitive) capacity assessment. It was supposed to be yesterday but because he was drowsy, they decided to wait and do it today. He's on subcutaneous fluids and this is very positional, but he won't let me touch it. He is resistive to care and is refusing washes. He hasn't had his bowels open for 4 days. He had several episodes of incontinence overnight, but I've managed to do an MSU. Nurse coordinator has arranged a discharge planning meeting for Friday at 1430. His next of kin is his nephew.

from *The Invisible Work of Nurses* (Allen, 2015) study, which has been lightly edited for pedagogical purposes and to protect patient identities. I have not added explanations for the terms and abbreviations used; understanding these is an important part of the sensemaking work involved in CTM. Read through Transcript 10.1 to familiarise yourself with the content and imagine yourself in this context. The transcript is reproduced in the Care Trajectory Management Workbook (see Evolve website) if you wish to highlight or annotate issues as you work through the exercises.

APPLYING THE CARE TRAJECTORY MANAGEMENT FRAMEWORK TO NURSING PRACTICE

This section considers the application of the CTM Framework to nursing practice.

Trajectory Awareness

Trajectory awareness is the first CTM Framework practice pillar and forms the foundations for CTM. Developing trajectory awareness involves reflexively monitoring and making sense of patient trajectories as they progress and encapsulating this understanding into a care trajectory narrative. While typically started through the nursing admission processes, it is the nursing handover which is the primary site for care trajectory narrative sharing and generation. Trajectories are always on the move and nursing handover is an opportunity to review and revise these understandings. Exercises 10.1–10.3 focus on trajectory awareness competencies development. Return to Transcript 10.1 to do the exercises. You can record your answers in the Care Trajectory Management Workbook (see Evolve website).

EXERCISE 10.1

Read through the medical ward handover and for each patient in your caseload; highlight and make a note of the salient elements you will need to refer to for the purposes of organising care.

EXERCISE 10.2

Review your caseload notes from Exercise 10.1 and create a second list of any issues which are ambiguous or unclear, and which require further sensemaking work.

EXERCISE 10.3

For each of the uncertainties you have identified, develop a plan for how you will resolve the issue.

EXERCISE 10.4

Return to the handover for the patients in your caseload and select the information that needs to be shared with other participants involved in the patient's care.

EXERCISE 10.5

Review your answers to Exercise 10.4 and document how and in what format you would communicate with each actor and explain the rationale for the communication strategies you have described.

At the end of these exercises, you should have a plot summary for the trajectory narrative of each of the patients in your caseload, and a plan of action for addressing any aspects of patients' care which are uncertain.

Trajectory Working Knowledge

Trajectory working knowledge is the second practice pillar in the CTM Framework. It refers to the processes of knowledge sharing through which nurses communicate with the various participants involved in a care trajectory. This entails identification of information that it is necessary to share for the purposes of trajectory management and translation of the pertinent elements of a trajectory narrative so that the right information is shared in the right format with the right people. Exercises 10.4 and 10.5 focus on trajectory working knowledge competencies development. Refer to Transcript 10.1 to do these exercises. You can record your answers in the Care Trajectory Management Workbook (see Evolve website).

At the end of these exercises, you should have identified the information requirements of the wider healthcare team and applied the skills of perspective taking and translation in thinking through your communication strategy.

Trajectory Articulation

This section considers the application to practice of the third pillar of the CTM Framework: trajectory articulation. Throughout this book, a large part of the discussion and the case study examples have focused on CTM in the context of individual patients, and the first of the exercises (Exercise 10.6) continues in this vein. However, with notable exceptions—such as intensive care—nurses work with multiple patients. Working with a caseload amplifies the complexity of the CTM work. Not only is the nurse required to make sense of and understand the trajectory of each of the individual patients under their care, but they must also be able to organise and prioritise activity across the caseload. The final exercise in this section (Exercise 10.7) is designed to develop skills in prioritising care. Return to Transcript 10.1 as suggested earlier to do the exercises. You can record your answers in the Care Trajectory Management Workbook (see Evolve website).

EXERCISE 10.6

For each patient in your caseload, identify the tasks that need to be organised, noting any potential temporal constraints, and who is responsible for the activity.

EXERCISE 10.7

Review your list of actions identified in Exercise 10.6 and rank them in order of priority.

At the end of these exercises, you should have a trajectory management plan for your caseload, which builds on the communication strategy developed in Exercises 10.4 and 10.5 and the activities identified for the purposes of clarifying trajectory awareness in Exercises 10.1–10.3. Collectively, these should orient you to the matters of concern for the purposes of CTM. These can be expressed as questions which act as useful prompts for practice:

- Information: What do I need to know?
- Communication: Who do I need to communicate with and how?
- Action: What do I need to do and in what order?

KEY CARE TRAJECTORY MANAGEMENT ACTIVITIES

Throughout this text, I have argued that CTM is a way of perceiving, understanding and acting that is woven through the fabric of everyday nursing practice and interspersed with clinical and unit management work. There are, however, certain activities in which the practices of CTM are at their most concentrated. This section focuses on these critical moments of healthcare practice.

Managing Transitions

This section considers the skills and competencies involved in managing transitions of care. As outlined in Chapter 9, the management of transitions is a central component of CTM. Before going any further, complete Exercise 10.8. Return to Transcript 10.1 to do this exercise. You can record your answers in the Care Trajectory Management Workbook (see Evolve website).

Transitions are a ubiquitous feature of nursing work. Transcript 10.1 is based on real-life data, and the number of transitions of care in this caseload is quite striking. Having completed Exercise 10.8, it should also be evident that in addition to being ubiquitous, care transitions are variable (Allen, 2015). In this example they include managing transfers of care for investigations (CT scan), an internal ward transfer, transfer from hospital to primary care and home care and planning for discharge. There is also reference to a patient who has been transferred from another ward. This list is by no means exhaustive, and it reflects activity on a medical ward in the UK National Health Service (NHS). Consider surgical settings and the work involved in managing the movement of patients from the ward to the operating theatre and back again, or the actions of community nurses, often allocated a specific clinical task, but who routinely review the stability of home care environments for meeting care needs following discharge from hospital, or the work of school nurses responsible for managing interfaces with educational, health and social care organisations.

While they are highly variable, all transitions have retrospective and prospective elements. They look back and require a summary of the relevant trajectory details from the transferring department about the history of the trajectory to date. They look forward and orient to the information that is necessary to facilitate the patient's onward trajectory or referral. In the language of TMT, this entails translation of the patient from the work object of one service into the work object of another. Transitions are managed in different ways; some involve face-to-face handover, others might involve a telephone conversation, others require complex multidisciplinary planning process, but all typically involve formal documentation—whether paper or digital. In other words, they are sociomaterial arrangements.

Documents have an important role in mediating the management of transition processes. They specify the information requirements of the receiving service and any actions and arrangements that are necessary to enable it to fulfil its functions. The information required by the receiving service may be quite different from the information required to support care in the transferring service, but

EXERCISE 10.8

Return to the handover and identify all those patients where reference is made to transitions of care.

EXERCISE 10.9

Imagine you are caring for Donald Evans (Bed 14) and have been asked to make a referral to Foxton Community Hospital. What information is required to support a safe transition? Remember, you may not have all the information necessary for this task in the handover.

it has been requested for a reason. Some services generate structured referral forms, which stipulate their requirements in detail, and may only need items to be ticked off by the referring service, such as the surgical checklist considered in Chapter 7 (Domain Assumption 4: Activities Have a Sociomaterial Distribution). Other documents are less structured and their success in mediating the transition of care hinges on the skills of the nurse in recognising the information requirements of the receiving service, which includes attending to how the person's needs may be impacted by the environment of care. The unified assessment documentation referred to in Chapter 9 (Box 9.4) was an example of an unstructured form. Whether structured or unstructured, managing transitions depends on the nurse adopting the perspective of others and undertaking the necessary actions to translate the patient into an object of their practice. Not all systems are well designed, and in pressurised conditions it may be tempting to regard the task as irritating 'paperwork', but if this is the only mechanism of knowledge sharing, or the only point of reference once the conversation about the patient has ended, then the consequences of getting this wrong can be serious. Exercise 10.9 focuses on these translational skills. Refer to Transcript 10.1 to do this exercise. You can record your answers in the Care Trajectory Management Workbook (see Evolve website).

Beyond knowledge translation, the management of transitions also typically involves articulation work to ensure the patient has everything required to support their needs during and following any transfer of care. Managing transitions encompasses attending to the material arrangements required to support the transition: equipment, information, medications, preparation of the patient. It also includes consideration of whether the transition arrangements cohere. For example, does the carer understand how to support medications management, are medications dispensed in a form that the person can take, and does the community nursing team have the information and the materials required to manage a specialist wound? Finally, managing transitions entails consideration of temporal factors so arrangements are aligned and available when needed—for example, the patient and/or family is prepared, equipment or medications ordered, services notified and transport organised.

The matters of concern for each aspect of articulation clearly depend on the transition in question, but as a rule of thumb, attending to the three facets of articulation should serve as a prompt to ensure everything has been attended to:

- Material: What material arrangements are needed?
- Integrative: Are the arrangements integrated?
- Temporal: Is everything lined up for when it is required?

Use this structure to complete Exercise 10.10 while referring to Transcript 10.1. You can record your answers in the Care Trajectory Management Workbook (see Evolve website).

While many transitions are highly routinised and the requirements of the receiving department are well specified, others can be infinitely more complicated and require extensive planning. Discharges from hospital are some of the most complex transitions of care, particularly in circumstances where the discharge destination is tentative. Organising transitions of care when a trajectory is still evolving, and outcomes are uncertain, is profoundly challenging. Consider

EXERCISE 10.10

Imagine you are caring for Lionel Black (Bed 15). List the activities required to ensure all the arrangements are in place to enable discharge.

EXERCISE 10.11

You have been asked to organise and attend the discharge planning meeting for Hugh Thomas (Bed 16). While a time has been scheduled for the meeting and Hugh's nephew has confirmed that he can attend, the coordinator has asked you to arrange the attendance of other key participants.

First, review the details of Hugh Thomas' trajectory from the handover extract.

Second, list all members of the team who ideally should attend the discharge planning meeting.

Third, review your list and select the team members who are essential attendees, and those whose perspectives and knowledge could be fed into the meeting without them having to attend in person.

Fourth, assuming that only essential team members will be in attendance, what key information is it necessary for the nurse to assemble and understand before the meeting?

You can record your answers in the Care Trajectory Management Workbook (see Evolve website).

EXERCISE 10.12

Reflection

Think about a practice area with which you are familiar and list the transitions for which nurses are responsible. Which work well and why? Which work less well and why? Which aspects of these processes would you change and in what way?

the examples of Edward Murphy (Chapter 7, Case Study 7.1) and Rosa Jackson (Chapter 3, Case Study 3.2), where there were disagreements between the healthcare team and family about the most appropriate arrangements. Settling upon transitional arrangements in complex cases often requires a dedicated planning meeting and nurses have a central role in leading these events. The final exercise in this section concerns the organisation and management a discharge planning meeting. Refer to Transcript 10.1 to do Exercise 10.11. Please download Template Exercise 10.11 to record your answer.

This section has focused on the CTM work involved in care transitions. Transitions of care are extraordinarily variable, ranging from highly routinised predictable arrangements to complex transitions which are inherently unstable. Some of the arrangements for managing transitions work well, but many do not. With increased professional awareness of, and confidence in, CTM expertise, nurses are well placed to initiate these kinds of service improvements (Exercise 10.12).

OPTIMISING INFRASTRUCTURES OF CARE

CTM is concerned with ensuring that all elements that support an individual's care and treatment are available when required. A fundamental way in which this can be achieved is by optimising the match between the needs of the person with the resources available in the care environment. The CTM activities involved in organising the infrastructures of care were considered in Chapter 9 (see Material Articulation). In this section we consider in greater detail two core activities: bed management in the acute sector and stabilising care arrangements in the community.

Matching Patients With 'Beds'

In the acute sector, clinical care is typically organised into specialist areas designed to meet the needs of specific patients. In this context, a 'bed' is much more than a comfortable place on which to lay one's head; it is associated with facilities, expertise, staffing establishments, infrastructure, technologies, materials and people. Research demonstrates that being in the right bed is beneficial for patients (Bucknall et al., 1988; Dunn, 2001; Mayor, 2005; Sanderson et al., 1990); consequently, matching the needs of people with the most appropriate 'bed' is an important moment of CTM.

EXERCISE 10.13

You are working as the ward coordinator. The medical bed manager informs you that there is a bed crisis in the hospital. The Emergency Department is overwhelmed, new cases are expected, and there is an urgent need to admit three new patients to release capacity. The bed manager has established that Lionel Black (Bed 15) is due to be discharged today and asks whether he can be moved to the Discharge Lounge while awaiting transport home. They also inquire whether the discharge plans of any other patients could be brought forward to today. Review the handover caseload and consider how you would manage the bed manager's request and account for your decision.

EXERCISE 10.14

You are informed that the new patient will require a single room. There are three single rooms on the ward. At present, these are occupied by Martin Blakemore (Bed 4), David Lister (Bed 13) and Donald Evans (Bed 14). Are any of these patients suitable to be moved into the main ward areas? Provide an explanation for your answer.

Contemporary healthcare systems are under considerable pressure, and patients can be admitted to a ward which is not designed for their care (often referred to as outliers), be moved within or between wards or have discharge planning processes accelerated to generate capacity. This is particularly the case in publicly funded healthcare systems (Alameda and Suárez, 2009). Patients categorised as outliers have increased length of hospital stay (Stylianou et al., 2017), and can challenge the skills of nurses (Cheung et al., 2020). Discharge planning processes and CTM are more challenging when patients are assigned to wards not designed for their care and treatment and may be disrupted when people move between clinical areas (Walford, 2002).

While nurses in the acute care sector are often employed in dedicated bed management roles, responsibility for bed management has become part and parcel of every nurse's role. Assigning people to the right bed with all the resources this brings has important implications for the quality, safety and efficiency of patient care. Accordingly, the ability to match patients with the right beds is an important nursing skill. These decision-making moments are often occasions in which expertise in balancing the care of individuals with the care of populations is brought into sharp relief (see Chapter 3: Complexity 7: Healthcare Requires Balancing the Needs of the Individual With the Needs of the Many) (Allen, 2015). Exercises 10.13 and 10.14 focus on these skills. Refer to Transcript 10.1 to do these two exercises. You can record your answers in the Care Trajectory Management Workbook (see Evolve website).

Stabilising Community Care Arrangements

Infrastructures of care in the community are often finely balanced arrangements. They can be quickly disrupted by a small change in one element of a patient trajectory, with negative consequences for patients and families, often leading to avoidable admissions to hospital. This is a particularly pertinent issue in older people, whether living permanently in residential facilities or their own homes. In this context, creating the conditions that optimise CTM entails reflexive monitoring of the match between an individual's needs and the arrangement in the environment of care and intervening to adjust and stabilise these arrangements as required. This might involve the gradual withdrawal of support as the person recovers from an acute episode, intervening to avert a crisis and prevent admission to hospital, and a whole range of tinkering and adjustments in between, as in the example of Cynthia in the previous chapter (see Case Study 9.1). Exercise 10.15 focuses on the practices involved in stabilising home care arrangements. Please refer to Transcript 10.1 to do this exercise. You can record your answers in the Care Trajectory Management Workbook (see Evolve website).

EXERCISE 10.15

In discussion with his wife, it was agreed that David Lister (Bed 13) could be cared for at home. He was discharged with a package of care which included morning and evening visits from a social carer to assist with his hygiene needs. The community nursing service was asked to call to change a leg dressing. Mrs Lister agreed to support David's medication management.

For the purposes of this exercise, imagine that you are the community nurse making a visit to attend to David's leg dressing. On arrival at the home, you are greeted by Mrs Lister, who is distressed, as her husband is very unwell and has been agitated overnight. She is tired and has slept little.

Mrs Lister directs you to the bedroom where the social carer is carrying out a bed bath. The social carer explains that David's condition has deteriorated quickly in 24 hours. This morning, he was very drowsy and unable to walk to the bathroom; he was also incontinent of urine on several occasions overnight. The carer is struggling to manage David alone, and so you assist her to finish the bed bath. While attending to David's hygiene needs, you discover a small sacral pressure ulcer, but there is no home care hospital bed and no provision for pressure relief.

Once you have made David comfortable, you discuss the situation with Mrs Lister. She is determined to honour David's wishes to remain at home at the end of his life and she believes that with some additional support she will be able to manage.

What adjustments need to be made to David's care arrangements to enable him to remain at home?

This section has focused on the skills involved in matching patient needs with care infrastructures. Securing a match would be relatively straightforward in a stable world, but healthcare systems and patient trajectories are far from stable. In the next section we will focus on approaches to assessing potential trajectory complexity, to be better prepared for such contingencies.

ASSESSING CARE TRAJECTORY COMPLEXITY

This section considers the factors which have the potential to make an individual's CTM more complex. Developing an awareness of the sources of complexity in patient's trajectories should not be taken to imply that it is possible to rationalise care, rather the intent is to facilitate a proactive approach to anticipate and manage potential challenges and reduce the risks of trajectories spinning out of control to become, what Strauss et al. (1985) call, cumulative mess trajectories.

The seven complexities of healthcare work (see Chapter 3) impact on trajectories of care to create different sources of complexity. These include diagnostic uncertainty; unstable care needs; disagreements between the health and social care team and family carers; the size and familiarity of the health and social care team; social issues, psychosocial factors; cognitive factors, financial factors; and legal factors (Allen, 2018). Identifying the potential sources of trajectory complexity requires a systematic approach to assessment, in much the same way as the nursing assessments that underpin care planning.

The sources of trajectory complexity arise from both individual and organisational factors. An individual may have an uncertain diagnosis or unstable care needs which compound trajectory management. Additional sources of complexity also stem from the clinical environment. For example, CTM in outlier patients is more difficult, as nurses may lack familiarity with patient requirements and relationships with the wider health and social care team may be more challenging. Assessments of care trajectory complexity should capture individual patient factors as well as organisational factors. Exercise 10.16 focuses on trajectory assessment skills. Before progressing

EXERCISE 10.16

Review your patient caseload.
First, list all the factors that have the potential to increase care trajectory complexity.
Second, reach an overall complexity assessment on a 5-point scale of 1 (low) to 5 (high). Third, think about the actions necessary to mitigate these risks.
If you wish, you can use examples from your own clinical practice for this exercise.
You can record your answers in the Care Trajectory Management Workbook (see Evolve website).

with this exercise, you may find it useful to refresh your understanding of the seven sources of healthcare complexity (see Chapter 3), as well as referring back to Transcript 10.1.

Assessments of trajectory complexity are not currently a routine feature of nursing practice, but there is a strong argument for why they should be. Beyond their value in informing care planning, the systematic measurement of CTM activity has the potential to generate two important sources of data. First, regular assessment of CTM complexity in the patient population produces data on the volume and complexity of CTM in the nursing workload, which can be included in workforce planning decisions (see Chapter 6: Care Trajectory Management Is Not Captured in Nursing Workload Measurement Systems). Second, there is the potential to generate insights into features of the organisational and clinical environment that may be compounding the complexity of CTM work, and which may be amendable to improvement, to reduce the burdens in the nursing workload (see Chapter 6: Nurses Sustain Faulty Systems Rather Than Intervening to Address Underlying Issues). This is clearly aspirational thinking, but as future leaders of the profession, it is important to think ahead to the work as it could be.

TALKING CARE TRAJECTORY MANAGEMENT

An important motivation for writing this book, indeed for undertaking *The Invisible Work of Nurses* (Allen, 2015) study, was to develop a language with which to describe and explain a central element of the nursing function that has hitherto had no name. The final exercises in this section (Exercises 10.17–10.19) focus on using the language of CTM and TMT to describe and advance

EXERCISE 10.17

Return to the handover data extract and your answers to Exercise 10.1. Imagine you have just finished reviewing your trajectory narrative notes following handover, and you are assessing the needs of the patients in your care, scrutinising the clinical notes and checking information on the computer. A first-year medical student asks what you are doing. Explain the care of the patients in your caseload using the language of the CTM Framework.

EXERCISE 10.18

You have been asked to contribute to a working group to inform the development of a new digital information system. How might you use your understanding of CTM to make the case for incorporating into the new system functions which support this work?

EXERCISE 10.19

You have been approached by the quality improvement manager to contribute to a service review. How might you make the case for using TMT as a framework for understanding the work as it is done, in advance of the development of an improvement plan?
Tip: It might be helpful to revisit Chapter 8 before you answer this question.

EXERCISE 10.20

Reflection

Revisit your account of your first experience of a healthcare setting as a student (see Chapter 3, Exercise 3.1). How has your knowledge of healthcare systems and CTM impacted on your understanding of the feelings you have described here?

nursing practice. Return to Transcript 10.1 to do these exercises. You can record your answers in the Care Trajectory Management Competencies Professional Development Assessment Framework in the Care Trajectory Management Workbook (see Evolve website).

Looking Back and Looking Forward

As you reach the end of this text, you should now have a good understanding of the organisational complexity of healthcare work and different approaches to tackling the challenges of organisation and coordination. You have learnt about the application of complexity science to healthcare, and how this offers new ways of thinking about some the intractable challenges of healthcare quality and safety, and the importance of attending to the practices and creativity of staff in enabling organisations to function despite the unpredictability of the work. You have learnt that CTM is an important source of organisational resilience in healthcare systems, and you now have the theoretical and conceptual resources with which to describe and explain this core component of nursing practice. Most of the exercises in the final chapter have focused on the primary care trajectory function, and the organisational knowledge that begins with the care of patients. But it is these skills and competencies that provide the foundations for advanced nursing practice in management and leadership roles. This includes being able to identify when CTM is masking system dysfunction, identifying the underlying issues and intervening to bring about improvements. It includes leading the implementation of new services (Krone-Hjertstrøm et al., 2021) and responding to healthcare crises as illustrated by the nursing response to the COVID-19 pandemic (Brunelli et al., 2021; Jackson and Nowell, 2021; Jónsdóttir et al., 2022; Kuijper et al., 2022). With a critical mass of nurses able to speak the language of CTM and share their professional vision, we create the opportunities for advances in practice, research and development, and elaboration of the theory, which will enable the profession to fully realise its contribution to contemporary healthcare systems (Exercise 10.20).

For the Journey...

The skills and competencies that underpin CTM are complex and need to be developed along the novice to expert continuum. The aim of this textbook was to provide the sensitising concepts and resources to accelerate the acquisition of these skills along the career pathway, support reflexive learning in clinical placements and encourage an acceptance and recognition of this work as a central pillar of nursing's professional identity. As you come to end of the book, review the CTM competencies summarised in Table 10.1 and identify three CTM professional development needs and a plan for achieving these. Enjoy the journey.

References

Alameda, C., Suárez, C., 2009. Clinical outcomes in medical outliers admitted to hospital with heart failure. Eur. J. Intern. Med. 20, 764–767.

Allen, D., 2004. Re-reading nursing and re-writing practice: towards an empirically-based reformulation of the nursing mandate. Nurs. Inq. 11 (4), 271–283.

Allen, D., 2015. The Invisible Work of Nurses: Hospitals, Organisation and Healthcare. Routledge, London and New York.

Allen, D., 2018. Care trajectory management: a conceptual framework for formalising emergent organisation in nursing practice. J. Nurs. Manag. 1, 4–9. doi:10.1111/jonm.12645.

Allen, D., Purkis, ME., Rafferty, AM., Obstfelder, A., 2019. Integrating preparation for care trajectory management into nurse education: competencies and pedagogical strategies. Nurs. Inq. 26 (3), e12289. doi:10.1111/nin.12289.

Bourdieu, P., 1980. The Logic of Practice. Stanford University Press, Stanford.

Brunelli, V.N., Beggs, R.L., Ehrlich, C.E., 2021. Case study discussion: the important partnership role of Disability Nurse Navigators in the context of abrupt system changes because of COVID-19 pandemic. Collegian 28 (6), 628–634.

Bucknall, C.E., Robertson, C., Moran, F., Stevenson, R.D., 1988. Management of asthma in hospital: a prospective audit. Br. Med. J. (Clin. Res. Ed.). 296, 1637–1639.

Cheung, J., West, S., Boughton, M., 2020. The frontline nurse's experience of nursing outlier patients. Int. J. Environ. Res. Public Health. 17, 5232. doi:10.3390/ijerph17145232.

Dunn, K.W., 2001. Standards and Strategy for Burn Care. https://www.britishburnsassociation.org/wp-content/uploads/2017/07/NBCR2001.pdf (Accessed 8 December 2022).

Goodwin, C., 1994. Professional vision. Am. Anthropol. 96 (3), 606–633.

Jackson, J., Nowell, L., 2021. The office of disaster management' nurse managers' experiences during COVID-19: a qualitative interview study using thematic analysis. J. Nurs. Manag. 29 (8), 2394–2400.

Jónsdóttir, H., Sverrisdóttir, S.H., Hafberg, A., Ómarsdóttir, G., Ragnarsdóttir, E.D., Ingvarsdóttir, S., et al., 2022. 'There was no panic' – nurse managers' organising work for COVID-19 patients in an outpatient clinic: a qualitative study. J. Adv. Nurs. 78, 1731–1742. doi:10.1111/jan.15131.

Krone-Hjertstrøm, Norbye B, Abelsen, B, Obstfelder, A., 2021. Organizing work in local service implementation: an ethnographic study of nurses' contributions and competencies in implementing a municipal acute ward. BMC Health Serv. Res. 21 (840), 840. doi:10.1186/s12913-021-06869-4.

Kuijper, S., Felder, M., Bal, R., Wallenburg, I., 2022. Assembling care: how nurses organise care in uncharted territory and in times of pandemic. Sociol. Health Illn. 44 (8), 1305–1323.

Mayor, S., 2005. Stroke patients prefer care in specialist units. Br. Med. J. 331, 130.

Sanderson, J.D., Taylor, R.F., Pugh, S., Vicary, F.R., 1990. Specialized gastrointestinal units for the management of upper gastrointestinal haemorrhage. Postgrad. Med. J. 66, 654–656.

Strauss, A., Fagerhaugh, S., Suczet, B., Weiner, C., 1985. The Social Organization of Medical Work. University of Chicago Press, Chicago, IL.

Stylianou, N., Fackrell, R., Vasilakis, C., 2017. Are medical outliers associated with worse patient outcomes? A retrospective study within a regional NHS hospital using routine data. BMJ Open 7, e015676. doi:10.1136/bmjopen-2016-015676.

Walford, S., 2002. Unexpected Medical Illness and the Hospital Response. Models of Emergency Care. University of Warwick, Warwick, UK.

Suggested Reading

Bed Management

Allen, D., 2015. Inside 'bed management': ethnographic insights from the vantage point of UK hospital nurses. Sociol. Health Illn. 37 (3), 370–384.

This paper examines one element of the care trajectory management role: bed management. There is relatively little research on everyday bed management practices and the paper engages with a previously published paper in the journal to show how, notwithstanding designated organisational roles designed for this purpose, bed management in contemporary healthcare systems has become the business of all nurses. Rather than the rational, centrally controlled processes espoused by policymakers, bed management is a distributed activity, best described as 'match making'. Here 'rationality' is not found in a centralised plan; rather, it is tied to the local situation in which nurses make the necessary accommodations and adjustments to balance demands with resources.

McGarry, J.R., Pope, C., Green, S.M., 2018. Perioperative nursing: maintaining momentum and staying safe. J. Res. Nurs. 23 (8). doi:10.1177/1744987118808835.

This study centres on the work of perioperative nurses and highlights the need for nurses to balance their responsibility for managing patient flows and delivering safe care.

Managing Transitions

Allen, D, 2015. The Invisible Work of Nurses: Hospitals, Organisation and Healthcare. Routledge, London and New York.

Chapter 5, 'Passing the Baton, Parsing the Patient' (pp. 108–131), describes and explains the work of nurses in managing transitions of care.

CTM Competencies

Allen, D., Purkis, M.E., Rafferty, A.M., Obstfelder, A., 2019. Integrating preparation for care trajectory management into nurse education: competencies and pedagogical strategies. Nurs. Inq. 26 (3), e12289. doi:10.1111/nin.12289.

This paper articulates the core competencies that underpin care trajectory management, but also outlines different pedagogical strategies for embedding preparation for practice into nursing curricula.

CTM and the Wider Nursing Role

Jackson, J, Anderson, J.E., Maben, J., 2021. What is nursing work? A meta-narrative review and integrated framework. Int. J. Nurs. Stud. 122, 103944. doi:10.1016/j.ijnurstu.2021.103944.

Jackson et al. report on a review of research on nursing work, including care trajectory management. It is useful resource for reflecting on the relationship of care trajectory management and the wider nursing role.

Chapter 1

Why has organising work had a bad press in nursing?
Organising work in nursing is often conflated with excessive paperwork and ineffective bureaucracy. There is ample evidence that the administrative processes in contemporary healthcare systems increase the burdens of work and do not always contribute positively to the quality of patient care. While these are very real issues, they should not distract attention from the importance of documentation in ensuring that patient care is coordinated and how nurses fulfil this function.

What is professional vision?
Professional vision refers to the distinctive ways of seeing a field which reflects practice concerns.

What is tacit knowledge?
Tacit knowledge refers to knowledge that cannot be articulated.

What is explicit knowledge?
Explicit knowledge refers to knowledge that can be articulated and shared.

How is theory useful in nursing practice?
Theory has value as it offers frameworks of understanding to illuminate, talk about and share nursing practice. Nurses already draw on a wide range of theories to inform their clinical practice, but no such theories exist in relation to the organisational components of the nursing role.

What are the changes that have occurred in healthcare that have created the need for care trajectory management?
Healthcare systems have become increasingly complex. This is a result of technological developments and advances in medical treatments, increased specialisation of the healthcare workforce and changes in disease patterns which has resulted in the growth in the prevalence of long-term conditions with many patients having more than a single problem. Collectively, these features make care processes unpredictable and the arrangements for ongoing support at home, challenging to maintain.

Chapter 2

Why is care trajectory a preferrable term to patient pathway?
Patient pathways have value in showing how care processes are organised for specific conditions, but they do not capture the unpredictable qualities of healthcare experienced by many patients and have less value in patient populations whose needs are too complicated or unpredictable to fit into a single plan of care. As patient populations increasingly present with complex conditions, great swathes of activity lay outside the reach of formal pathways.

What elements are included in the concept of a care trajectory?
The concept of a trajectory of care refers to all the elements involved in meeting the needs of the patient and the impact of this work on all those involved and the organisation of these processes.

Which elements of nursing practice does care trajectory management refer to?
Those aspects of nursing practice concerned with the coordination and organisation of patient care.

Chapter 3

What are the seven complexities of healthcare work?
Healthcare is a work of many hands, it is technologically complex, it is people work, illness and recovery are unpredictable, the needs of individuals must be balanced with the needs of the many, it entails multiple institutional logics, and it is distributed work.

Why did Melia argue that simply measuring the tasks involved in patient care missed many of the activities and skills involved in hospital nursing?
Melia argued that hospitals have turbulent work environments and nursing activities reflect the demands of managing the environment in addition to the work of patient care.

What does it mean to describe healthcare as a 'collective endeavour'?
Healthcare is not the work of a single individual; it involves input from a wide range of professions, technicians, the patient and their family.

What is burden of treatment theory?
Burden of treatment theory is a theory which acknowledges, describes and explains the demands placed on patients and their families in managing treatment regimens. It has been developed as an alternative to behavioural change approaches, for understanding nonadherence and focuses on the burdens of treatment.

What is meant by 'technology' in understanding healthcare work?
The term 'technology' has a broad application in healthcare research. It includes everyday devices, medicines, highly sophisticated equipment and assistive technologies.

Why can the term 'teamwork' be a misleading description of healthcare?
The notion of teamwork is misleading in healthcare because for much of the time, the work is widely distributed, clinicians work largely independently and understanding of the patient is fragmented between different members of the healthcare team.

What is the cumulative complexity model?
The cumulative complexity model was developed by Shipee et al. to describe and explain how patients' care and treatment can become increasingly complicated as individual factors interact with each other in dynamic ways.

What is biographical disruption?
The term 'biographical disruption' was introduced into the literature by Bury, to refer to the impact of illness on the person's sense of self.

What is biographical flow?
The notion of biographical flow builds on ideas about biographical disruption, to draw attention to the impacts of an individual's illness on the wider family.

What is an institutional logic?
An institutional logic refers to a set of assumptions, beliefs and values that drive activity. Multiple institutional logics can coexist in a single setting. Sometimes these work in concert, sometimes they can conflict.

What is a complex adaptive system?
A complex adaptive system refers to systems that have dynamic qualities which cannot be reduced to their individual parts. The application of these ideas to understanding healthcare is growing in the face of the challenges of intervening in services to bring about improvements in healthcare quality and safety.

Chapter 4

What are the origins of rational–linear approaches to organisation?
Rational–linear approaches to organisation originate in the classical management theories of the 19th century and which were responsible for the introduction of the assembly line and processes of standardisation.

What are the origins of emergent approaches to organisation?
Strauss and their team developed the negotiated order perspective, which was one of the first process models of organisation. It was based on their empirical research in healthcare settings.

What is the primary difference between rational–linear and emergent approaches to organisation?
Rational–linear approaches to organisation privilege structures and processes and understand organisation as a top-down process. Emergent approaches to organisation underline the fluid and unpredictable qualities of organisation and understand organisation as arising from the actions taken from the bottom up in creating order out of complexity. Whereas rational–linear approaches treat organisations as if they were a machine, emergent approaches emphasise the dynamic qualities of organisations.

Why are rational–linear approaches an attractive solution to organisational challenges?
Rational–linear approaches align with accepted cultural models of legitimate ways of organising activity.

What image from ornithology best depicts rational–linear approaches to organisation?
Geese flying in formation.

What image from ornithology best depicts emergent approaches to organisation?
A murmuration of starlings.

Why does healthcare require both rational-linear and emergent approaches to organisation?
Healthcare is a complex system and without structures, they would be utterly chaotic. Certain activities can usefully be managed by rational–linear approaches; these are typically processes which have a degree of predictability and regularity. However, other areas of healthcare work require more responsive approaches to organisation tailored to individual needs.

Why do Greenhalgh and Papoutsi argue that the workarounds and muddling-through that keep the show on the road are not footnotes in the story, but its central plot?
This is a statement of the importance of the emergent organising practices of staff at the frontline.

Chapter 5

What is a Prevention of Future Deaths Report?
A report produced by UK coroners following an inquest if it appears that there is a risk of other deaths occurring in similar circumstances.

What is the difference between proximal and distal factors in understanding service processes?
These terms indicate how far the cause of an issue of concern is from the centre of a safety or quality failure. Proximal factors have a close relationship to the failure, whereas distal factors are more removed.

What is root cause analysis?
A systematic methodology used to understand the system and process issues contributing to critical incidents.

What is resilience engineering?
An approach to understanding safety which attends to how systems adapt to changes in conditions to continue to function.

What is organisational resilience?
A property of organisational systems which enable them to function despite unpredictable changes in the work.

Chapter 6

In what way is care trajectory management functionally invisible work?
Care trajectory management is functionally invisible work because it is work that can be seen but it is taken for granted.

What is professionalisation?
The process through which occupations develop the qualities which indicate their status as a recognised profession to claim societal rewards for their members.

What is jurisdiction?
This term was introduced into the literature by the sociologist Andrew Abbott, and it refers to the scope and the rationale for a profession's claim to expertise to a particular area of work.

How have professionalisation processes in nursing rendered care trajectory management invisible?
Nursing's professionalisation project was predicated on a professional identity centred on nurses' caregiving role. In this context, and in the face of service pressures on the nursing workload, the organisational elements of nursing work have been interpreted as a distraction from the caring function.

What is the tragedy of adaptability?
This term was coined by Wear and Hettinger. It refers to the processes through which the responsive interventions of frontline staff in addressing the unpredictable qualities of the work can also mask underlying system issues, which remain unaddressed.

Chapter 7

What is a grounded theory?
A grounded theory is a theory derived from empirical data, rather than abstract reasoning.

What is a middle range theory?
Middle range theories tend to focus on a circumscribed issue or problem, rather than large-scale phenomenon.

Which two processes are associated with a process view of organisation?
The two processes associated with the process view of organisation are 'negotiations' and 'sensemaking'.

What is an artefact?
An artefact is any object produced by human beings; 'objects' can be material or cognitive.

What is the difference between a formal and an informal artefact?
Formal artefacts are official recognised in organisations, informal artefacts are developed by staff to support their work, but they are not formally sanctioned.

What is meant by 'affordance' in descriptions of artefacts?
Affordance refers to the qualities and characteristics of an artefact which determines what it can do and how it can be used.

Chapter 8

What is a project in Translational Mobilisation Theory (TMT)?
The project is the unit of analysis in TMT, and it refers to the activity of interest.

What is a strategic action field in TMT?
This strategic action field refers to the context in which a project takes place, features of which condition how work is done.

What are the four features of a strategic action field that impact on how an activity is accomplished?
These are structures (fixed points and stable features, such as roles and departments), organising logics (the norms, priorities and values that drive activity), interpretative repertoires (cognitive and meaning-making resources), materials (physical infrastructure, expertise, technologies).

What are mechanisms of mobilisation in TMT?
In TMT mechanisms of mobilisation refer to *how* a collective activity is organised and accomplished.

What is object formation?
This refers to the processes through which actors in a strategic action field draw on interpretative resources to create the objects of their practice.

What is translation?
This refers to the mechanisms which enable the objects of practice in a collective activity to be shared between participants and these different understandings accommodated.

What is articulation?
Articulation refers to the mechanisms which ensure that all the elements required to support an activity are aligned when they are required; it is the work that makes the work, work.

What is reflexive monitoring?
This refers to the mechanisms through which actors in a collective activity monitor and review the progress of projects to coordinate their efforts.

What is sensemaking?
This term refers to the processes through which actors make sense of complex organisational circumstances and create order in achieving and accounting for action.

Chapter 9

What is trajectory awareness?
Trajectory awareness refers to the understanding developed by nurses of all the elements involved in a trajectory care, and their interrelationships, as these evolve over time.

What are the three mechanisms involved in developing and maintaining trajectory awareness?
Maintaining trajectory awareness involves the mechanisms of reflexive monitoring, sensemaking and object formation.

What is trajectory working knowledge?
Working knowledge refers to the practices through which nurses draw on their trajectory awareness, which is encapsulated in trajectory narratives, to ensure flows of communication between trajectory actors.

What is the mechanism involved in developing trajectory working knowledge?
Trajectory working knowledge involves translation; this mechanism entails taking the perspective of others and translating information into a format oriented to the requirements of the recipient.

What is trajectory articulation?
Trajectory articulation refers to the practices involved in ensuring that all elements necessary to meet patient need are lined up in the right place at the right time; this involves both proactive action and interventions and responsive adjustments to changing conditions.

What are the three forms of trajectory articulation?
There are three types of trajectory articulation: temporal (ensuring actions happen at the right time), integrative (ensuring that actions and decisions are joined up) and material (attending to the infrastructure, technologies and expertise that support care). These are frequently combined in practice.

Chapter 3

EXERCISES 3.2–3.8
GARETH WILLIAMS CASE STUDY 3.1

EXERCISE 3.2

List all the people, departments or services involved in Gareth William's acute care from the onset of the stroke to his discharge home. Don't worry if you do not know all the precise role titles.

Meryl Williams
Emergency medical response call handler
Emergency medical response despatch officer
Paramedics and emergency medical response staff
Administrative staff
Radiographers
Radiologist
Specialist nurse stroke coordinator
Bed manager
Thrombolysis team
Speech and language therapist
Ward nurses
Ward medical staff
Physiotherapist
Occupational therapist
Pharmacist
Dietician
Laboratory staff
Catering staff
Domestic staff
Portering staff
Primary care doctor
Primary care nurse
Stroke support group
Physiotherapist (private)

EXERCISE 3.3

List all the technologies involved in Gareth's care in hospital and at home. Let your imagination roam freely; don't just focus on sophisticated equipment, consider everyday technologies too. What functions do these technologies perform? How do these technologies impact on Gareth Williams' care?

Here's an indicative list, which is far from exhaustive.
Monitoring equipment (on the scene, in the ambulance, in thrombolysis and in continuing care on the ward; this could be electronic or manual, intermittent or continuous)
Emergency response vehicle and associated technology
Stretcher
Manual handling equipment
Medications
CT scanner
Blood test technology (needles, syringes, bottles, laboratory equipment)
Hospital bed
Medical record, nursing record, physiotherapy record, occupational therapy record, dietician record, primary care record
ICT
Charts and forms for recording clinical care
Thrombolysis technologies
Urinal
Bedpan
Shower, bath, toilet
Pens
Paper
Telephone
Hospital bleep
Shower
Assistive technologies
Infusion technologies

EXERCISE 3.4

It is 4 days after Gareth Williams was admitted to hospital with an acute stroke. His care and progress will be reviewed at the ward round. Return to the list you generated in Exercise 3.2 and identify which actors are currently involved in Gareth's care. For each actor identified, write down which aspects of Gareth's care they are knowledgeable about. Now, reflect on your experiences of a typical ward round and consider who, from your list, is likely to be present for the event. How is the knowledge of absent participants built into discussions and decision making?

Actors currently involved in Gareth's care include:
Medical staff—detailed understanding of medical conditions and physiological indicators
Ward nurses—understanding of Gareth's care needs and emotional well-being, relational knowledge of Meryl and her ability to support Gareth after discharge and overview of Gareth's trajectory of care
Dietician—understanding of the dietary requirements for the management of diabetes, insights into Gareth's reaction to and understanding of his diabetes diagnosis
Speech and language therapist—understanding of Gareth's speech and swallowing issues
Physiotherapist—understanding of Gareth's mobility issues
Occupational therapist—understanding of the organisation and layout of Gareth's home and where assistive technologies may have value
Meryl Williams—understands impact of stroke on Gareth and can possibly anticipate how he will approach rehabilitation
Pharmacist—understands Gareth's medications management
A typical ward round includes only medical and nursing staff. Occasionally, it may involve the physiotherapist and the occupational therapist, but rarely the dietician, pharmacist, speech and language therapist or family member. Nurses are often the means through which the knowledge of absent actors is built into discussion. We also know that it can be difficult for nurses to attend ward rounds, which raises serious issues about the comprehensiveness of the information available to medical staff in making decisions.

EXERCISE 3.5

Identify any aspects of Gareth's illness and recovery that made, or had the potential to make, his trajectory of care unpredictable.

These might include his newly diagnosed diabetes requiring changes to diet; his weight, which may have impacted on mobilisation and skin integrity; the impact of the stroke on Gareth's identity; and his depression.

EXERCISE 3.6

Review Case Study 3.1 to consider how the 'people' element of Gareth Williams' care impacted on his recovery trajectory.

Gareth refused to have handrails fitted out of concern for his house-proud wife. The couple refused support from the Community Resource Team as they considered that they could manage, but then Garth became depressed and lacked the motivation to continue with his rehabilitation exercises without support and ended up paying for this privately.

EXERCISE 3.7

After discharge from hospital, and despite his wife's efforts, Gareth was reluctant to follow a diabetic diet to manage his blood glucose levels. This was related to his depression. What logics are involved in the compromises that were reached in managing this scenario in the immediate period following discharge?

The compromises that were reached were informed by a logic which privileged Gareth's mental health and physical rehabilitation over his need to lose weight and manage his diabetes. This was a short-term strategy and was possible as Gareth's diabetes was mild.

EXERCISE 3.8

Return to Case Study 3.1 and review Gareth Williams' care from the point of admission home. How has his care been shaped by health services resource management, and prioritisation processes?

The emergency medical services arrived quickly as stroke care is time-critical and the algorithms used by the call handlers in managing the call would have categorised this as a high-priority call.
When Gareth realised that he needed a physiotherapist to support rehabilitation at home, there was a waiting list for the community service, and so he elected to pay privately for this service. Gareth was fortunate in having the resources to fund his care; this option is not available to everyone.

CT, computed tomography; ICT, information communication technology.

Chapter 4

EXERCISE 4.3

You have been approached to contribute to the development of an end-to-end pathway for stroke management. Return to Case Study 3.1 (Chapter 3) and think about the different stages of Gareth Williams' trajectory of care. Are there aspects of care and treatment that might usefully be managed by a pathway? Are there aspects of care and treatment where a pathway has less value? Explain the reasons for your answers.

The early treatment of stroke is time-critical and standardised. This makes the initial trajectory of care very well suited to pathway use. But stroke impacts people in different ways and rehabilitation trajectories are more variable. In conditions of variability, standardised pathways have less value.

Chapter 5

EXERCISE 5.1

Review the code book of subthemes identified by Leary et al. (2021). Considering what you have learnt about proximal and distal factors, select which categories of concern might be attributed to failures of care coordination or organisation and note the reasoning behind your answer.

Category of Prevention of Future Death Report Concern Subtheme	Categorise EACH ITEM √ = poor coordination was a contributory factor ? = poor coordination may have been a contributory factor X = poor coordination was not a contributory factor	Give the Reason for Your Answer
Deficit in skill or expertise	X	This is assumed to refer to individual clinical skills deficits.
Failure to deviate from algorithmic care or policy when harmful or inappropriate	?	This could be understood as an example of inappropriate reliance on rational-linear models of organisation when the situation required an emergent or responsive approach.
Failure to be aware of, follow or implement evidence-based guidance	?	This could be understood as a failure to follow a standardised approach when it was required.
Misprescribing	X	This is assumed to refer to clinical skills deficits or errors.
Misdiagnosis	X	This is assumed to refer to clinical skills deficits.
Unnecessary or inappropriate investigations or care	?	This is most likely to indicate clinical skills deficits, but incomplete information could have been a factor, and so poor coordination may be implicated in this example.
Inappropriate equipment usage	?	Coordination failure could be a distal factor in this example, if inappropriate equipment was used because of equipment unavailability.
Human error during procedures	X	This example clearly relates to human error.
Care (including investigations and assessments) not done	?	Coordination failure could be a contributory factor here, but failures of this kind might arise from staff shortages or capacity issues too.

Continued

Cont'd

Category of Prevention of Future Death Report Concern Subtheme	Categorise EACH ITEM √ = poor coordination was a contributory factor ? = poor coordination may have been a contributory factor X = poor coordination was not a contributory factor	Give the Reason for Your Answer
Failure to report concerns to the organisational leaders or regulator	X	This is not a coordination failure.
Reactive culture	?	Coordination failure could be a contributory factor here, where 'reactive culture' points to a failure to anticipate need. It's important not to confuse the importance of responsive forms of organisation with a reactive culture. The former is a necessary element to evolving trajectories of care. The later is a consequence of planning failures.
Ergonomics and design of equipment	X	Coordination is not a factor in this example.
Equipment failure	X	Coordination is not a factor in this example.
ICT unsuitability/failure	X	Coordination is not a factor in this example, although ICT issues can impact on coordination.
Failure to share records in ICT platforms across organisations	√	Clearly a failure to coordinate knowledge and information; but such issues are not always within the power of frontline staff to address. Staff often must work around infrastructural shortcomings, which adds to the volume of coordination work.
Unable to access records (paper or ICT)	√	This example is clearly a failure to coordinate knowledge and information, but such issues are not always within the power of frontline staff to address. Staff often must work around infrastructural shortcomings, which adds to the volume of coordination work.
Care (including investigations and assessments) significantly delayed	?	Poor coordination could certainly be a factor here, but capacity issues are often responsible for delays in care, investigations and assessments.
Uncoordinated/unmanaged care	√	A self-evident example of poor coordination.
No/poor assessment of care needs	√	A self-evident example of poor coordination. Care cannot be coordinated if needs have not been assessed.
No or insufficient care plan	√	A self-evident example of poor coordination. Care cannot be coordinated if needs have not been assessed and a plan agreed.

No or insufficient advice on self-care	√	A self-evident example of poor coordination, remember your learning on the role of patients in trajectories of care.
Inappropriate care setting (no or inadequate assessment)	?	Whilst not caused by poor coordination per se, as you will learn later in this book, allocating patients to the correct care setting is an important mechanism of ensuring that their needs are met.
No or inappropriate medicines management (polypharmacy/over prescribing/oversupply of medication)	√	Failure to assess how individual medications act and interact is a form of coordination failure.
Failure/refusal to communicate with other team members or agencies	√	A self-evident example of poor coordination.
Failure/refusal to communicate with carers/families	√	A self-evident example of poor coordination.
Poor/unsuitable environment	?	Whilst not caused by poor coordination per se, as you will learn later in this book, allocating patients to the correct care setting is an important mechanism of ensuring that their needs are met.
Contracting or financial disputes	X	Coordination is not a factor in this example.
Failure to provide care/treatment due to demand management policy/strategy	?	The requirement to introduce demand management may arise because of capacity issues, which in turn may reflect organisational failures relating to patient flow. There are likely to be lots of confounding issues in this example.
Reorganisation of services	?	Here, the issues could reflect coordination failures of new structures.
No or insufficient learning form internal investigations	X	Coordination is not a factor in this example.
Concerns about postmortem procedures	X	Coordination is not a factor in this example.
Medicines unavailability	X	This is most likely a supply issue, but failures to plan and order medications for when they are required could be a contributory factor here.
Out-of-date applications ('apps')	X	Coordination is not a factor in this example.
Failure to document care	√	Documentation of care is central to coordination of effort.
Retrospective documentation both after the fact (question of reliability) or with alleged intent to deceive	X	Coordination is not a factor in this example.
Language or cultural misunderstanding	X	Coordination is not a factor in this example.
Inconsistent terminology	√	Inconsistent terminology can be a cause of coordination failure, as it leads to communication difficulties and mitigates the development of a shred perspective.

Continued

Cont'd

Category of Prevention of Future Death Report Concern Subtheme	Categorise EACH ITEM √ = poor coordination was a contributory factor ? = poor coordination may have been a contributory factor X = poor coordination was not a contributory factor	Give the Reason for Your Answer
Missing notes/documents	?	Not caused by coordination failure, but highly likely to contribute to it.
Staff stress	X	Coordination is not a factor in this example.
Refusal to treat	X	Coordination is not a factor in this example.
Dishonesty	X	Coordination is not a factor in this example.
Failure or absent leadership	X	Coordination is not a factor in this example.
Misuse of equipment	X	Coordination is not a factor in this example.
Inappropriate use of resources (i.e., police)	?	This is not a coordinating failure as such. But it is indicative of failures in understanding of roles and responsibilities, which is an essential prerequisite for coordination.
Lack of policy/guidance	X	Coordination is not a factor in this example.
Regulatory issues	X	Coordination is not a factor in this example.
Untraceable staff	X	Coordination is not a factor in this example.
No response to coroner	X	Coordination is not a factor in this example.
Equipment missing	X	A supply issue, possibly; but regular audits are essential to ensure that equipment is available when it is required.
No or insufficient staffing	X	Coordination is not a factor in this example.
High workloads	X	Coordination is not a factor in this example.
Unable to recruit	X	Coordination is not a factor in this example.
Lack of staffed beds	?	This is clearly a capacity issue, which may reflect failures in managing patient flow.

ICT, information communication technology.

Leary, A., Bushe, D., Oldman, C., Lawler, J., Punshon, G., 2021. A thematic analysis of the Prevention of Future Deaths reports in healthcare from HM coroners in England and Wales 2016–2019. J. Patient Saf. Risk Manag. 26(1), 14–21. doi:10.1177/2516043521992651.

EXERCISE 5.2

Review the proximal and distal factors contributing to safety threats during hospital discharge identified by Waring et al. (2016) and identify the safety threats at discharge in which the coordination or organisation of care was *not* a contributory factor. Explain the reasons for your answers.

Category of Threat	Examples	Explanation	Safety Threat Is Not Related to Coordination
Proximal 'contributing' factors Definition: Actions, conditions or triggers that were seen as the primary or immediate cause of a safety incident	Assessment of patient	This refers to disagreements between the team as to whether the patient is ready for discharge, and uncertainty about whether medical fitness was a sufficient basis on which to progress a discharge.	Poor coordination is a contributory factor.
		Other issues related to the failure of the acute sector to address secondary health problems, which could be consequential for the success of discharge plans.	Poor coordination is a contributory factor.
	Completion of tests	Participants described that some tests ordered during discharge planning were not completed. Some patients were discharged before tests results were back.	Poor coordination is a contributory factor.
	Ordering and use of equipment	Bureaucratic processes for ordering.	Not an obvious coordination failure, but a factor which impacts on coordination.
		Uncertain lines of responsibility across health and social care providers.	Poor coordination is a contributory factor.
		Delays in equipment installation.	Not an obvious coordination failure, but a factor which impacts on coordination and could indicate poor planning.
		Poor education of patients and families on equipment use.	Poor coordination is a contributory factor.
		Different technologies used in hospital and community context.	Not an obvious coordination failure, but which could impact on coordination of transitions of care.
	Provision and management of medicines	The prescriptions of medications to take home were rushed, inaccurate or incomplete.	Not a coordination failure as such, but an error that impacts on coordination.
		Inadequate checking of medications before discharge.	Not a coordination failure as such, but an error that impacts on coordination.
		Patients and families reported poor information on medication management.	This is a coordination failure.
	Follow-up care and monitoring	Hospital participants highlighted issues arising from inadequate support provided in the community, including the limited involvement of the primary care doctor following discharge from hospital.	This is a coordination failure.

Continued

Cont'd

Category of Threat	Examples	Explanation	Safety Threat Is Not Related to Coordination
Distal latent factors Definition: Distal factors included those underlying or system-level issues that participants commonly described while explaining why a safety event might have occurred and which were understood as an enduring or cross-cutting issue that impacted upon care quality through shaping the context in which more proximal factors occurred.	Discharge planning	There was no standardised process for discharge planning and 'a general sense of complexity, confusion and poor integration between the different health and social care systems of work that was seen as conditioning many of the problems of care planning'	This is a coordination failure.
		There were challenges in involving all team members in planning meetings 'this meant that concerns about patient mobility, cognition or lifestyle factors were not fully considered [...] [and] on-going discharge plans would often be incomplete or missing important detail'.	This is a coordination failure.
	Referral processes	Many problems were associated with referral processes to community and social services.	This is a coordination failure.
		Paperwork associated with referral processes was perceived to be excessive.	Not a coordination failure as such, but a factor which could contribute to poor coordination and make transfers of care more difficult.
		Accessing patient information to make a referral was difficult when information was spread across multiple record-keeping systems.	Not a coordination failure as such, but a factor which could contribute to poor coordination and make transfers of care more difficult.
	Discharge timing	Participants highlighted the problem of premature discharge on the one hand, and delayed discharge on the other.	This is a symptom of the challenges of planning for discharge when patient trajectories are still evolving, as well as the difficulty of predicting the impact of the home environment.
		It could be difficult to agree the timing of discharge with the work schedules of acute and community providers.	This is partly about capacity and partly about coordination.
	Resources constraints	Participants highlighted the challenges of constraints on community resources which could delay discharge or create the conditions in which discharge arrangements were suboptimal.	This is a capacity issue, NOT a coordination failure.
	Organisational demands	Participants pointed to the pressures on acute hospital beds and patient flow and the constraints on the availability of social care provision in the community.	This is a capacity issue, NOT a coordination failure.

Waring, J., Bishop, S., Marshall, F., 2016. A qualitative study of professional and carer perceptions of the threats to safe hospital discharge for stroke and hip fracture patients in the English National Health Service. BMC Health Serv. Res. 14(16), 297.

Chapter 8

EXERCISES 8.1–8.10

What Is the Project?	Define the Scope of the Project	Ecology of People, Materials and Technologies
EXERCISE 8.1 Select an activity with which you have experience. This can be example from healthcare, but an activity from another context you are familiar with can be used for this exercise. Just make sure it is an activity that is dependent on collective effort that is people working together.	A multidisciplinary research study in healthcare funded by a research charity	The research team (qualitative researchers, health economist, statistician and clinical experts) The research protocol (formal statement of the study design and research instruments) Physical and technological infrastructure Research participants Funding body

Strategic Action Field

Structures
EXERCISE 8.2
Document the structures involved in your selected project of action.

Roles within the research team (chief investigator, collaborators, researchers), research participants (healthcare organisations, patients and healthcare staff), academic departments, funding body, ethics committees, research regulatory frameworks, research users (patients, public providers), wider research community.

Organising Logics
EXERCISE 8.3
Document the organising logics involved in your selected project of action; remember that these may be contradictory.

Most research is driven by common logics relating to the requirements of methodological and scientific rigor, research ethics and governance frameworks and the relevance and transferability of the study findings to clinical practice.
Within this overarching framework, however, different disciplines have their own logics. Qualitative social scientists are concerned with depth of understanding, accessing a full range of perspectives and the generation of empirically grounded concepts and theories; health economists are concerned with accurate costing of all inputs; and statisticians are concerned with identifying the appropriate and reliable outcome measures and generate robust data sets with sufficient power to undertake predictive modelling. Clinical team members may be more concerned with the practical implications and transferability of the research.
The success of an applied project hinges on the management of these different logics.

Interpretative Repertoires
EXERCISE 8.4
List the formal and informal interpretative repertoires involved in the project and how these shape how the activity is accomplished.

Depending on the study, these could include formal study design, different theoretical frameworks, economic models, statistical analyses, researcher interpretations.
Some studies begin with a theory which the research is designed to test (a deductive approach). Other studies develop theory from the analysis of empirical data (an inductive approach). Large studies may incorporate deductive and inductive elements.
Patient and publics bring their own interpretative repertoires to studies, which are drawn from user experiences.

Continued

Cont'd

What Is the Project?	Define the Scope of the Project	Ecology of People, Materials and Technologies
Materials **EXERCISE 8.5** Document the infrastructure, technologies and materials involved in the project of interest.	Projects are also shaped by the availability of materials and resources that condition the possibilities for action. These include the amount of funding, the ICT infrastructure (computers, word processor, data analysis software, reference managers, email; Teams/Zoom), office space, storage facilities, audio-recorders and the availability of data (costs of services, routinely collected outcomes data).	

Mechanisms

Object Formation **EXERCISE 8.6** Document the objects of practice involved in the project of interest.	The research protocol is the overarching object of practice and fulfils an important function of enrolling all relevant actors into the project, agreeing to the research question and study design, negotiating roles and responsibilities (chief investigator, principal investigators, research managers, workstream leads, clinicians, researchers, and patient/public representative—and advisory and/or steering group membership) and identifying the resources required and how these are distributed. While methodologies and techniques are to some extent standardised, these must be adapted to the technical and logistical requirements of the project, the relationship between elements of the research must be formalised, and research aims must be aligned with the possibilities for investigation. Undertaking the research involves the creation of new objects of practice: data analysis plans and associated artefacts (data extraction templates, interview schedules, coding frames), research ethics materials (research protocol, study information sheets, consent forms) and communication resources (project website, business cards, newsletters, media launch and conference presentations).	
Translation **EXERCISE 8.7** Think about the translations that are necessary to enable participants to work together to accomplish the activity. These might not be linear processes as in the example of rescue trajectories; concentrate on key moments of communication between participants when one participant's interpretation and way of describing a situation need to be translated into the language of another to facilitate understanding or mobilise action.	Much health-related research involves collaboration between multidisciplinary teams, including different academic subject specialists, clinicians and patient or public representatives. Communicating across disciplinary boundaries can be challenging and there is a need to develop understanding among team members. This may not simply be a case of finding a common language but thinking about a problem in an entirely different way and working through the logic of this reformulation for the study. Participants in the research project may have different degrees of interpersonal familiarity; some may have worked together on previous projects, for others these relationships need to be developed de novo. These connections take time to develop and maintain, a factor rarely considered by research funding bodies, but it is essential that participants from different disciplinary backgrounds can work together around a common project.	

Articulation
EXERCISE 8.8

Think about those aspects of the project that need to be articulated and how this happens. What are the formal or informal mechanisms involved?

All projects have a chief investigator who has overall responsibility for the research. Large studies often include a study manager who organises and supervises adherence to regulatory processes (ethics committees and research and development departments), manages the budget and mediates relationships with the funders.

It is also quite common for there to be designated workstream leads within a study, particularly if they use mixed methods.

Oversight of a research project is formally managed through regular study management meetings. However, workstream members often meet more frequently to discuss operational issues and these are important occasions for articulating elements of the research, for example, if assumptions that were built into the study protocol do not align well with the reality in the field.

Large studies often have an independent steering group, which maintains oversight of overall study progress.

Reflexive Monitoring
EXERCISE 8.9

What are the processes through which participants monitor the status of an activity? Once again, this can be formal or informal, it can be at individual, team or system level, or include elements of each.

Research is an emergent activity, necessitating adjustments and revisions to the original plans. This is an acknowledged challenge for health services researchers, as the institutional context in which research projects are carried out is predicated on a biomedical model of science and demands high degrees of stability and centralisation.

Any changes to the study necessitate a restatement and approval of new structures and standards to bring these in line with the emerging nature of the research. Unsurprisingly, then, much of the reflexive monitoring, in the context of research projects, is driven by the need to ensure alignment with the formal study protocol and hinges on formal processes of mapping progress against an agreed plan of activity and reviewing efforts across different elements of the study to ensure coherence.

The funding body and steering group have a role here in monitoring progress against objectives and making critical decisions about the study's continuation in the face of delays in progress.

Sensemaking
EXERCISE 8.10

How do sensemaking processes impact on the project of interest and how is this distributed across participants?

Sensemaking is a central component of any research study. It includes the work of research staff in applying the study instruments to the data generation process, the work involved in applying a standardised coding framework to raw data, and it is involved in the interpretative efforts involved in exploring the relationship between data and theory and conceptual frameworks. In mixed-methods research, it is a central component in the work of synthesising data of different kinds.

ICT, information communication technology.

Chapter 9

EXERCISE 9.5

Use the CTM Framework to identify the TMT mechanisms of involved in Case Study 9.1. Imagine you are a qualitative researcher, analysing the data to locate evidence of the practice pillars and mobilisation mechanisms from the CTM Framework.

CASE STUDY 9.1 Cynthia's antibiotic management

The first lady we are visiting today is **'Cynthia', an elderly woman who has diabetes and memory problems. CCC explained that her diabetes is controlled with medication but that 'her blood sugars are all over the place'. The plan is to reduce the dose of diabetes medication.** CCC has been asked to go in and **'monitor things'. She explains that Cynthia has carers to assist with washing and dressing and they are allowed to prompt her to take her medications, but they are not allowed to give them to her. Her medications are managed through blister packs. (Blister packs are a technology for helping people to keep track of their medications. Medications are dispensed weekly and combined in a designated sealed compartment or bubble to be taken at specific times of the day.)**

Trajectory awareness

Reflexive monitoring

Trajectory awareness

We arrive at the flats where Cynthia lives and wait to be let in using the intercom system. On entry we are confronted by a wall of heat and CCC observes, 'crikey it's hot in here'. Cynthia is watching breakfast television and is still in her dressing gown. **CCC asks how she is, and Cynthia says she is not well as she has a 'water infection' and is 'feeling a bit sick'. Cynthia says that she has contacted her primary care doctor who is coming to see her today, but that she has also been seen by 'another doctor' who prescribed her more tablets.** She hands these to CCC; they are trimethoprim, an antibiotic used to treat urinary tract infections. Someone has written on the medication box that these tablets are to replace the evening maintenance dose of the same drug Cynthia regularly takes, and which is included in her blister packs. **CCC takes out a folder from the shelf under the television and reads through the notes. (This, I later found out, was the carers' folder.)**

Reflexive monitoring

Sensemaking

CCC: Here it says that on the 12th the doctor got them delivered but there's nothing here to say the trimethoprim was removed from the box. (The reference to 'box' in this utterance refers to a locked Dossett box, where Cynthia's medications are kept because of her memory problem, and which can only be accessed by the home carers.)

CCC is concerned and explains that there are several tablets in the blister packs to be administered at a given time and the carers are not able to remove the unwanted drug from the blister pack. Therefore, with the new prescription, the dose of trimethoprim Cynthia is receiving is too high which can cause renal failure. In addition, because of Cynthia's memory problems, all medications should be kept in the locked Dossett box. CCC explained that part of the problem was that Cynthia was being seen by out-of-hours primary care doctors who 'had only part of the picture' and would not appreciate some of the challenges with her memory or the practical challenges involved in her medication management. CCC suggests to Cynthia that she stops taking the trimethoprim.

Material and integrative articulation

CCC then makes a call to the home care agency to obtain information on the code to access the Dossett box to enable this to be shared with the out-of-hours primary care doctors so they can change the contents of her medications if necessary. She explains that the out-of-hours doctor has prescribed trimethoprim and someone has written on the medications box to omit the maintenance dose. **She confirms with the care agency that carers are not allowed to remove medications from the blister packs.**

Sensemaking

We return to the sitting room, and CCC then attempts to contact Cynthia's primary care doctor to discuss the issues with the out of hours team, but she learns that the doctor is seeing a patient. Initially, she says she will hold, but after a minute or so, she is informed that the doctor is likely to be 5 minutes or more and suggests that the doctor calls her back. CCC then turns attention to taking Cynthia's blood glucose reading which is the purpose of the visit. She spends some time searching her bag for reagent sticks. As she is searching, Cynthia turns to me and says: 'Don't get old dear'.	Integrative articulation

CCC, community care coordinator.

Chapter 10

EXERCISES 10.1–10.3

Caseload	EXERCISE 10.1	EXERCISE 10.2	EXERCISE 10.3
	Read through the medical ward handover and for each patient in your caseload, highlight and make a note of the salient elements you will need to refer to for the purposes of organising care.	Review your caseload notes from Exercise 10.1 and create a second list of any issues which are ambiguous or unclear, and which require further sense-making work.	For each of the uncertainties you have identified, develop a plan for how you will resolve the issue.
Bed 1: Mark Haven	Uncertain diagnosis; monitor pain and psychological impact on the patient, and prepare for discharge.	Pain status is uncertain, medication is uncertain, home circumstances and implications for discharge are also unclear.	Review pain and psychological impact with the patient and inform doctor; consultant prescription chart to ascertain pain medication: discuss home circumstances with the patient and consider plans for discharge.
Bed 2: Sebastian Turner	For transfer of care to Robinson Ward. Discharge documentation to be completed. Family uncertainty about ability to cope at home, social worker to be contacted to discuss package of care.	Uncertainty about home care package. Bed availability on Robinson Ward.	Contact social worker to discuss homecare package ahead of transfer of care. Confirm bed availability on Robinson Ward and when this will be available.
Bed 3: Kevin Potter	Wound clinic appointment (1430). Education about management of diabetes and diet.	Unsure how patient is to be transported to wound clinic and preparation necessary. Understanding of diabetes unclear?	Clarify transport arrangements for wound clinic. Talk to the patient about understanding of diabetes; consider referral to a dietician.
Bed 4: Martin Blackmore	CT scan at 2 PM; the family want to be present when sharing results.	Clarify whether Martin needs to be nil by mouth for CT scan.	Clarify when CT scan results will be available and inform the family about timing.

Continued

Cont'd

Caseload	EXERCISE 10.1	EXERCISE 10.2	EXERCISE 10.3
Bed 5: Brian Lowes	Discharge planning and assessments; ? stairs assessment; discharge planned for Thursday but ??? feasibility, ? review homecare package. Can bring bed downstairs, but daughter needs to be notified.	Clarify whether the stairs assessment been done and, if so, what was the outcome.	Clarify whether the physiotherapist has done a stairs assessment. Discussion with MDT members, Brian and daughter to assess feasibility of planned discharge date and home carer support needs.
Bed 6: Jackson Mitre	Chest X-ray, to be seen by neurology team.	Longer-term plans for care uncertain.	Discuss with Jackson and the MDT team the longer-term plans for care.
Bed 7: Norman Hollingsworth	? Feels fine and no issues	Can he be discharged? Has the course of antibiotics been completed?	Ascertain home situation and consider discharge.
Bed 8: Hamish Drew	Bypassing catheter, planning for home.	Discharge plans unclear. Reasons for bypassing catheter are unclear and the issue needs to be resolved.	Investigate reasons for bypassing catheter and address. Consider implications for discharge. Consider organising a discharge planning meeting.
Bed 9: Carlton Regis	To start 24-hour tape and 24 hour urine; locate acid, family concerned/dissatisfied.	Tests awaiting 'acid'.	Contact relevant department to obtain 'acid' to expedite 24-hour tests, keep Carlton and family informed.
Bed 10: Mohammad Kaif	Non-English speaker.	No clear plans indicated in handover.	Discuss longer-term plans with the medical team, discuss home circumstances with the family.
Bed 11: Ian Howells	Preparation for home, exercise tolerance test, warfarin, needs TTHs.	When is exercise tolerance test planned? Does Ian understand warfarin management requirements?	Check notes and contact relevant department. Discuss warfarin management with Ian.
Bed 12: Edward Logan	Review discharge plans, doctor's assessment required; plan for residential care?	Plans for discharge quite unclear, need to be clarified.	Speak to the MDT, Edward and Mrs Logan, to clarify discharge plans. Explain funding implications. Discuss homecare option with social worker.
Bed 13: David Lister	DNAR, meeting for the wife and the doctor re palliative care.	When is the doctor available to discuss care with David's wife?	Speak to the doctor to organise a meeting with Mrs Lister.
Bed 14: Donald Evans	DNAR; urgent referral to Foxton Community Hospital.	Referral is urgent, but it is unclear whether there is a bed available and whether this has been agreed with the patient and family.	Discuss referral to Foxton Community Hospital with the patient and son; establish bed availability at Foxton Community Hospital.

Bed 15: Lionel Black	Home today, TTHs done, book ambulance at 1300, check with dietician re. thickener, supply thickener to take home.	Are there any medical concerns about the incident in which Lionel coughed up blood?	Check the medical record and speak to the doctor if necessary re coughing up blood.
Bed 16: Hugh Thomas	Mobility? Cognitive assessment, discharge planning meeting 1430—nephew to attend, bowels not opened for 4 days.	Establish history of mobility. Could constipation account for decline?	Review notes and speak to nurses from Bluebell Ward; contact doctor re constipation.

CT, computed tomography; DNAR, do not attempt resuscitation; MDT, multidisciplinary team; TTHs, tablets to take home.

EXERCISES 10.4–10.5

Caseload	**EXERCISE 10.4**	**EXERCISE 10.5**
	Return to the handover for the patients in your caseload and select the information that needs to be shared with other participants involved in the patient's care.	Review your answers to Exercise 10.4 and document how and in what format you would communicate with each actor and explain the rationale for the communication strategies you have described.
Bed 1: Mark Haven	Inform doctors about pain so discharge planning can proceed.	This could be in person or over the telephone.
Bed 2: Sebastian Turner	Comprehensive handover required for Robinson Ward.	This will be written referral documentation and potentially verbal handover with nursing staff (in person or by telephone).
Bed 3: Kevin Potter	Potential referral to the dietician for diabetes management.	Telephone call and formal referral.
Bed 4: Martin Blackmore	Ensure doctors are aware of family wishes re CT results.	In person or by telephone.
Bed 5: Brian Lowes	Discuss Brian's needs with the social worker to establish whether he can have an increased care package. Full discussion with the MDT to review feasibility of discharge date.	This could be by telephone. This would require a meeting.
Bed 6: Jackson Mitre	Trajectory information for the neurology team.	This would be in the form of an appropriately designed trajectory narrative.
Bed 7: Norman Hollingsworth	Update on progress with medical staff so that discharge can be considered.	Document patient status in medical record, and update the doctor in person.
Bed 8: Hamish Drew	Discussion with doctor about his catheter. Discussion with MDT and family re discharge.	A focused discussion about the issues concerned, having first appraised the situation. This would require a meeting.
Bed 9: Carlton Regis	Keep family appraised of care plans.	Proactive face-to-face communication during visiting time or in response to inquiries.

Continued

Cont'd

Caseload	EXERCISE 10.4	EXERCISE 10.5
Bed 10: Moham-mad Kaif	Communicate uncertainty about long-term care to medical staff.	Face to face, and probably the kind of issue that is most suitably raised on the ward round.
Bed 11: Ian Howells	Request TTHs from doctor.	Request could be left in the doctors' job book if it is not urgent.
Bed 12: Edward Logan	Review discharge plans with the MDT, but particularly the social worker.	This would require an MDT meeting.
Bed 13: David Lister	Discuss the doctor's availability for a meeting with David Lister's wife.	In person—face to face or by telephone.
Bed 14: Donald Evans	Share information about Foxton Community Hospital with Donald and his family. Comprehensive handover for Foxton Community Hospital Staff.	In person—face to face or by telephone. This will be written referral documentation and supplementary verbal handover with nursing staff (most likely by telephone).
Bed 15: Lionel Black	Review thickener referral with the dietician.	Check the patient notes, but then a telephone call is sufficient to clarify this point.
Bed 16: Hugh Thomas	Ensure all MDT members are aware of discharge planning meeting.	Speak to key individuals, either in person or by telephone.

CT, computed tomography; *MDT,* multidisciplinary team; *TTHs,* tablets to take home.

EXERCISES 10.6–10.8

Caseload	EXERCISE 10.6	EXERCISE 10.7	EXERCISE 10.8
	For each patient in your caseload, identify tasks that need to be organised, noting any potential temporal constraints, and who is responsible for the activity.	Review your list of actions identified in Exercise 10.6 and rank them in order of priority.	Return to the handover and identify all those patients where reference is made to transitions of care.
Bed 1: Mark Haven	Plan for discharge when pain settles, establish home circumstances, organise doctor to write up TTHs.	Medium priority, which could become more urgent if beds are required.	Discharge.
Bed 2: Sebastian Turner	Completion of referral documentation for Robinson Ward. Establish homecare arrangements with the social worker.	High priority: if Robinson Ward has a bed. Ascertaining this information before transfer would be preferrable, but not essential.	Internal transfer to Robinson Ward.
Bed 3: Kevin Potter	Ensure arrangements are in place to attend wound clinic. Discuss diabetes management with Kevin. Contact dietician re diet.	Urgent, the appointment is at 1430. Important, but not urgent. Important, but not urgent, and contingent on the outcome of the discussion with Kevin.	Wound clinic.

Bed 4: Martin Blackmore	Establish whether Martin should be nil by mouth for his CT scan.	High priority; if Martin eats or drinks, this could result in the cancellation of the CT scan.	CT scan.
Bed 5: Brian Lowes	MDT discussion re feasibility of discharge. A dedicated meeting will take time to organise. It might be possible to initiate a discussion in routine meetings, or gather information from MDT members to feed into ward round.	Medium priority.	Planning for discharge.
Bed 6: Jackson Mitre	Ensure preparation for chest X-ray.	High priority, but not a large task.	Chest X-ray.
Bed 7: Norman Hollingsworth	Establish whether Norman can be discharged. A dedicated meeting will take time to organise. It might be possible to initiate a discussion in routine meetings, or gather information from MDT members to feed into ward round.	Medium priority, which could become more urgent if beds are required.	? Discharge.
Bed 8: Hamish Drew	Get the doctor to review catheter. Establish discharge plans. A dedicated meeting will take time to organise. It might be possible to initiate a discussion in routine meetings, or gather information from MDT members to feed into ward round.	Nonurgent. Medium priority, which could become more urgent if beds are required.	? Discharge.
Bed 9: Carlton Regis	Expedite 24-hour tests.	Medium priority.	
Bed 10: Mohammad Kaif	Clarify longer-term plans. This can be raised in routine team meetings.	Nonurgent.	
Bed 11: Ian Howells	TTHs to be written up.	Medium priority, which could become more urgent if beds are required.	Exercise tolerance test. Discharge.
Bed 12: Edward Logan	Clarify discharge plans. It might be possible to initiate a discussion in routine meetings, or gather information from MDT members to feed into ward round.	Medium priority, which could become more urgent if beds are required.	Discharge. ? Nursing home care.

Continued

Cont'd

Caseload	EXERCISE 10.6	EXERCISE 10.7	EXERCISE 10.8
Bed 13: David Lister	Arrange for the doctor to discuss discharge and palliative care options with David's wife.	Medium priority, which could become more urgent if beds are required.	Discharge and palliative care options.
Bed 14: Donald Evans	Discuss Foxton Community Hospital with Donald and his family. Contact Foxton Community Hospital to establish bed availability.	Urgent—to expedite planning.	Foxton Community Hospital.
Bed 15: Lionel Black	Book ambulance. Confirm whether the dietician has done thickener referral. Locate thickener for Lionel to take home. Confirm with the doctor that there are no concerns about the coughing incident.	All urgent tasks—discharge dependent and ambulance booked for 1 PM to align with home carers.	Discharge. Ambulance.
Bed 16: Hugh Thomas	Ensure team members are aware of discharge planning meeting.		Transferred from Bluebell ward.

CT, Computed tomography; *MDT,* multidisciplinary team; *TTHs,* tablets to take home.

EXERCISE 10.9

Imagine you are caring for Donald Evans (bed 14) and have been asked to make a referral to Foxton Community Hospital. What information is required to support a safe transition? Remember, you may not have all the information necessary for this task in the handover.

Review the handover transcript:

Staff Nurse 3: Bed 14 Donald Evans – 94. End stage COPD. He's DNAR now – as of yesterday. He told the doctors he wanted to die. The nephew is looking for a nursing home – Polar View, but there are four before him on the (waiting) list.

Staff Nurse 4: He's getting depressed and needs to be nearer to home for people to visit. So I think we should think about referring him to Foxton Community Hospital. Otherwise, he is going to die here which is not appropriate.

Information on Donald's medical history and recent care.
Information on Donald and the family's awareness of his prognosis.
Information on Donald's nursing care (psychological, hygiene, skin integrity, mobility, manual handling issues, falls risks, nutrition, and hydration, continence and management) and details on Donald's preferences which will enhance individualisation.
Information on Donald's medication management.
Information on next of kin and family contact numbers.
Information on Donald's DNAR status.
Information on Donald's known dietary preferences.
Information on any supportive technologies used for the purposes of Donald's care.
Information on any assistive technologies: eye glasses, hearing aid, prostheses, dentures
Relevant social history and interests.

EXERCISE 10.10

Imagine you are caring for Lionel Black (bed 15). List the activities required to ensure all the arrangements are in place to enable discharge.

Review the handover transcript:

Staff Nurse 3: Bed 15, Lionel Black. Going home today. TTHs dispensed. Nina could not book an ambulance yesterday as she was trying to get hold of the social workers to find out when the care package started. She called back at 5! So can we book an ambulance for 1 pm. His wife knows. All we need to do is to confirm with the dietician to see if she has done the referral for going home with thickener. We also need to send thickener with him as well. Oh, one more thing. During handover, his wife showed us fresh blood coming from his cough. It was in a tissue. He saw the doctor who was not concerned and thought it had just come from coughing.

Book ambulance for 1 PM.

Contact the dietician to confirm thickener referral.

Obtain thickener for Lionel to take home; ensure Lionel and his wife understand how this should be used.

Provide TTHs and ensure Lionel and his wife understand medications management. Provide written information if required.

Provide a sharps box if this is necessary.

Confirm arrangements for social carers and ensure Lionel and his wife are aware.

Assist Lionel to pack his belongings to take home.

Ensure all the material arrangements to support discharge are in place: handrails, walking frame, raised toilet seats, commodes, chair raises, bed.

Ensure ambulance crews can access the home.

TTHs, tablets to take home.

EXERCISE 10.11

You have been asked to organise and attend the discharge planning meeting for Hugh Thomas (bed 16). While a time has been scheduled for the meeting and Hugh's nephew has confirmed that he can attend, the coordinator has asked you to arrange the attendance of other key participants.

Review the handover transcript:

Staff Nurse 3: Bed 16 – Hugh Thomas – 86 – admitted with a chest infection and came to us from Bluebell Ward. They apparently said he was mobilising independently but with us when he mobilised to the toilet he was very unsteady and yesterday was very drowsy. So not sure what's going on there. We are just waiting for a (cognitive) capacity assessment. It was supposed to be yesterday but because he was drowsy, they decided to wait and do it today. He's on subcutaneous fluids and this is very positional, but he won't let me touch it. He is resistive to care and is refusing washes. He hasn't had his bowels open for 4 days. He had several episodes of incontinence overnight, but I've managed to do an MSU. Nurse coordinator has arranged a discharge planning meeting for Friday at 1430. His next of kin is his nephew.

List all members of the team who ideally should attend the discharge planning meeting.	Review your list and select the team members who are essential attendees.	Review your list and select the team members whose perspectives and knowledge could be fed into the meeting without them having to attend in person.	Assume that only essential team members will be in attendance. What key information is it necessary for the nurse to assemble and understand before the meeting?
Ward nurse who knows Hugh	Ward nurse	Nurse from Bluebell Ward	You could liaise with the nurses from Bluebell Ward to better understand Hugh's earlier trajectory.
Medical consultant	Nephew	Depending on the outcome of the report, it might be acceptable for the psychologist not to attend the meeting in person.	
Nephew	Medical consultant		The psychologist will provide a report, which can be discussed in advance of the meeting.
Physiotherapist	Social worker		
Psychologist (carried out cognitive capacity assessment)	Physiotherapist		
Nurse from Bluebell ward	Psychologist		
Social worker			

EXERCISE 10.13
You are working as the ward coordinator. The medical bed manager informs you that there is a bed crisis in the hospital. The Emergency Department is overwhelmed, new cases are expected, and there is an urgent need to admit three new patients to release capacity. The bed manager has established that Lionel Black (Bed 15) is due to be discharged today and asks whether he can be moved to the discharge lounge while awaiting transport home. They also inquire whether the discharge plans of any other patients could be brought forward to today. Review the handover caseload and consider how you would manage the bed manager's request and account for your decision.

There is no reason why Lionel Black cannot be moved to the discharge lounge if all the arrangements are in place for him to be safely discharged.
Other patients who have the potential for discharge include:
Bed 1: Mark Haven, who is young, and could be discharged if his pain settles.
Bed 5: Brian Lowes has a planned discharge, but the arrangements are complex and there is some uncertainty about their feasibility, so not suitable for escalation.
Bed 7: Norman Hollingsworth claims to be feeling fully recovered, and so discharge could be discussed with the doctor. Issues that would need resolving include planning for continuing his course of antibiotics, and clarifying Norman's home circumstances and any arrangements for his ongoing care.
Bed 8: Hamish Drew—there are plans for discharge, but there is also an ongoing issue with a urinary catheter, which presents risks for an escalated discharge.
Bed 11: Ian Howells—if the exercise tolerance test is satisfactory, he could be suitable for discharge assuming that TTHs could be prescribed and arrangements put in place for his Warfarin management.
Bed 14: Donald Evans—requires a transfer of care, which could be expedited if there is a bed available, transport can be organised, and Donald and his son agree.
The most obvious candidate is Mark Haven.

EXERCISE 10.14
You are informed that the new patient will require a single room. There are three single rooms on the ward. At present, these are occupied by Martin Blakemore (Bed 4), David Lister (Bed 13) and Donald Evans (Bed 14). Are any of these patients suitable to be moved into the main ward areas? Provide an explanation for your answer.

Donald Evans is at end of life and should not be moved.
David Lister is at end of life and should not be moved.
Martin Blakemore could be facing distressing news as the result of his CT scan, and so I would be disinclined to move him.
If it was possible to expedite Donald's transfer of care to Foxton Community Hospital with the agreement of the patient and family, then this could help generate the capacity required.

CT, Computed tomography.

EXERCISE 10.15
In discussion with his wife, it was agreed that David Lister (Bed 13) could be cared for at home. He was discharged with a package of care which included morning and evening visits from a social carer to assist with his hygiene needs. The community nursing service was asked to call to change a leg dressing. Mrs Lister agreed to support David's medication management.
For the purposes of this exercise, imagine that you are the community nurse making a visit to attend to David's leg dressing. On arrival at the home, you are greeted by Mrs Lister, who is distressed, as her husband is very unwell and has been agitated overnight. She is tired and has slept little.
Mrs Lister directs you to the bedroom where the social carer is carrying out a bed bath. The social carer explains that David's condition has deteriorated quickly in 24 hours. This morning he was very drowsy and unable to walk to the bathroom; he was also incontinent of urine on several occasions overnight. The carer is struggling to manage David alone, and so you assist her to finish the bed bath. While attending to David's hygiene needs, you discover a small sacral pressure ulcer, but there is no home care hospital bed and no provision for pressure relief.
Once you have made David comfortable, you discuss the situation with Mrs Lister. She is determined to honour David's wishes to remain at home at the end of his life and she believes that with some additional support she will be able to manage.
What adjustments need to be made to David's care arrangements to enable him to remain at home?

Consider insertion of an indwelling catheter if urinary incontinence continues to be a problem, given the sacral pressure sore.

Organise a hospital bed and pressure relieving mattress.

Review pain management.

Increase the social care package to three visits a day and two carers per call. Refer the case to the community palliative care nurses.

EXERCISE 10.16
Review your patient caseload.

First, list all the factors that have the potential to increase care trajectory complexity.

Second reach an overall complexity assessment on a 5-point scale of 1 (low) to 5 (high). Third, think about the actions necessary to mitigate these risks.

If you wish, you can use examples from your own clinical practice for this exercise.

Caseload	Care Trajectory Management Complexity Assessment	Overall Assessment 1 (Low)–5 (High)	Plan the Actions Necessary to Mitigate Risk
Bed 1: Mark Haven	Uncertain health status but not a cause of medical concern. Possible psychological anxiety about the pain and uncertainty about the underlying cause. Echo. Discharge to be planned.	2	Reassurance re cause of pain; review home situation and plan arrangements for safe discharge once pain has settled.
Bed 2: Sebastian Turner	Uncertain health status but planning for rehabilitation. Care team will change with internal transfer of care. Uncertainty about the social situation and continuing care arrangements at home. Patient is 'really vague'—poor cognition could impact on planning processes. Activity involved in transfer to Robinson Ward.	3	Clarify home situation with the social worker; comprehensive handover to Robinson Ward nurses to mitigate any disruptive effects of the transfer of care.
Bed 3: Kevin Potter	Newly diagnosed diabetes. In addition to the ward, Kevin is under specialist care of wound team; could be considered for referral to the dietician. Long-term resident in a nursing home. Nonengagement with diabetes and dietary requirements. Discharge to nursing home.	2	Patient education re diabetes and referral to dietician; prepare for discharge to nursing home where Kevin is known to the team.
Bed 4: Martin Blackmore	Health status is uncertain. Potential for bad news following scan, family wish to be with the patient. Preparation of patient for CT scan and transitional arrangements between ward and scanner.	3	Minimal planning possible until the results of the CT scan are known, potential for new tests to be required, lots of psychological support in coping with unwelcome or uncertain diagnosis.

Continued

Cont'd

Caseload	Care Trajectory Management Complexity Assessment	Overall Assessment 1 (Low)–5 (High)	Plan the Actions Necessary to Mitigate Risk
Bed 5: Brian Lowes	Coordinate OT and physio assessments. Continuing care needs to be reviewed. For discharge home, but complex plan.	4	Maintain oversight of OT and physio assessments and review their implications for discharge; maintain communications with daughter; liaise with social worker re. continuing healthcare needs; plan for discharge with comprehensive package of support liaising with community care providers as necessary.
Bed 6: Jackson Mitre	Uncertain and unstable health issues, and long-term comorbidities. Extended care team, which includes neurology. Chest X-ray to prepare for. Careful discharge planning required.	4	Work needs to be done to make sense of this case and think about the long-term plans for care and discharge.
Bed 7: Norman Hollingsworth	Acute diarrhoea which has now resolved. Need to plan for discharge.	1	Review home arrangement and plan for discharge.
Bed 8: Hamish Drew	Longstanding health issues, bypassing catheter. Need to plan for discharge.	4	Plans for discharge—likely to need a complex package of care to support continuing care needs, investigate and resolve issues re. catheter.
Bed 9: Carlton Regis	Uncertain health status. Anxiety re. health condition and family concern about treatment. Absence of acid for urine test leading to delays in test to inform diagnosis. 24-hour tape and 24-hour urine to plan.	3	Support for patient and family as tests are undertaken to reach a diagnosis, organisation of tests.
Bed 10: Mohammad Kaif	Chest pain, but managed with GTN. Support family to help mitigate language issues. Uncertainty about longer-term plan.	3	There is no obvious plan in this case, mobilising the team to agree a plan will ensure sufficient time to put in place discharge arrangements.
Bed 11: Ian Howells	Clear diagnosis (PE) and treatment. Exercise tolerance test to prepare for. Discharge with plans in place for warfarin management.	2	Prepare for exercise tolerance test, plan for discharge home, organise arrangements for warfarin management, patient education and materials for warfarin management.

Bed 12: Edward Logan	Acute episode of constipation, but evidence of long-term support needs. Patient and wife requested residential home placement. Finance could be an issue in funding residential home care. Discharge to be planned, but timing and destination uncertain.	3	Handover indicates that both patient and wife agree about the desirability of a residential placement. Identifying a suitable care home and organising the finances to support this can be time-consuming. But the main issue from a nursing perspective is to reflexively monitor these arrangements and be prepared to mobilisation action when required.
Bed 13: David Lister	COPD and DNAR, transitioning to palliative care. Review of home circumstances to inform discharge plan. Support for David and Mrs Lister in adapting to prognosis. Consideration of palliative care options (hospice or home) and planning accordingly.	5	Organise and participate in discussion between the doctor and Mrs Lister to discuss David's prognosis and long-term care plan; agree on the discharge destination and plan accordingly.
Bed 14: Donald Evans	End-of-life care for end-stage Chronic Obstructive Pulmonary Diease. Donald is becoming depressed; urgent need to transfer his care to a facility nearer his friends and family. Urgent transfer to community hospital required.	5	Contact Foxton Community Hospital to ascertain bed availability; meet with Donald and nephew to consider Foxton Community Hospital; expedite rapid discharge if indicated.
Bed 15: Lionel Black	For discharge home. For discharge management; ambulance to be booked, dietician referral, arrange thickener coordinate and integrate elements.	4	Book ambulance, ensure all elements required to support discharge are assembled; check with doctor about cough.
Bed 16: Hugh Thomas	Uncertain and unstable health status. Uncertain cognitive capacity, capacity assessment planned. Transferred from another ward.	5	High levels of uncertainty in this case; initial priority for the nurse is to ensure all relevant information is available for the discharge planning meeting.

COPD, Chronic obstructive pulmonary disease; *CT,* computed tomography; *DNAR,* do not attempt resuscitation; *GT,* glyceryl trinitrate; *OT,* occupational therapy; *PE,* pulmonary embolism.

Agency The ability to think and act in social systems which expresses an individual's power.

Artefact An object, whether this is material, cognitive or virtual, which is made by human beings.

Articulation Derived from the work of Strauss et al., articulation is a mechanism in Translational Mobilisation Theory which refers to the work processes in projects of collective action that ensure the integration and coordination of the work.

Care trajectory Derived from the work of Strauss et al., care trajectory refers to the unfolding of a patient's health and social care needs, the total organisation of work carried out over its course and the impact on those involved with that work and its organisation.

Care trajectory management Derived from the work of Allen to refer to the role of nurses in mobilising, coordinating and organising the relationships involved in trajectories of care.

Care Trajectory Management Framework Developed by Allen, and building on the Translational Mobilisation Theory, the Care Trajectory Management Framework provides a structure and language to explain nursing's care trajectory management function.

Care trajectory narrative Derived from the work of Allen, this concept refers to narratives which encapsulate the core features of an evolving trajectory of care, and which are used by nurses to coordinate activity.

Complexity science The study of complex systems which cannot be reduced to an understanding of their constituent elements.

Distributed cognition Derived from the work of Hutchins, this term is used to describe situations in which knowledge is dispersed over a community of individuals and external artefacts, rather than being represented in individual brains.

Emergent organisation An approach to organising in which order is understood as developing from the interactions between participants as they make sense of and manage situations, conundrums and unexpected occurrences in their work.

Habitus Developed by Bourdieu, this concept refers to the socially acquired habits, skills and dispositions which shape how individuals perceive and react to the social world around them.

Institutional logics A set of assumptions, beliefs and values that guide activity and are reflected in material practices, work cultures and symbolic representations.

Integrative articulation In Translational Mobilisation Theory, integrative articulation refers to the action undertaken to ensure decision-making is joined up and the individual elements in a trajectory of care cohere.

Interpretative repertoires In Translational Mobilisation Theory, interpretative repertoires denote the formal and informal cognitive artefacts and meaning making resources available within a strategic action field.

Material articulation In Translational Mobilisation Theory, material articulation refers to the practices required to ensure the availability, organisation and alignment of the physical resources involved in a trajectory of care.

Materials In Translational Mobilisation Theory, materials denote the physical infrastructure, technologies and concrete resources within a strategic action field which condition the performance of an activity and the sociomaterial distribution of work.

Negotiation A term derived from symbolic interactionist sociology which refers to the processes through which actors interpret and act in situations and in so doing create social order.

Object formation A mechanism in Translational Mobilisation Theory, this refers to the processes through which participants involved in a project of collective action use the interpretative and material resources within a strategic action field to create the objects of their practice.

Object of practice A socially constructed focus of interest that reflects the work purposes of an individual actor in a system of work.

Organisational resilience How a complex system adjusts its function to sustain its operation despite the unpredictable qualities of the work.

Organising logics In Translational Mobilisation Theory, organising logics refer to those elements of a strategic action field—norms, values, priorities—that drive how things are done in a project of action and shape its purpose.

Perspective-taking The practice of taking the perspective of others and understanding their information requirements.

Professional vision Derived from the work of Goodwin, professional vision refers to the socially organised ways of seeing and understanding an area of practice aligned with the interests or concerns of a social group.

Professionalisation The activities through which an occupation seeks to secure societal legitimacy through the development of skills, identities and norms associated with the traits of a recognised profession.

Rational–linear organisation The dominant approach to organisation underpinned by engineering and management science, which privileges planning, standardisation, guidelines and structural solutions to the challenges of organisation.

Recipient design When information or an utterance is designed with the needs of the recipient in mind.

Reflexive monitoring Derived from research on implementation led by May and Finch, reflexive monitoring is a mechanism in Translational Mobilisation Theory which refers to the processes through which actors collectively or individually appraise and review the progress of an activity.

Sensemaking Derived from the work of the social psychologist Weick, sensemaking is a mechanism in Translational Mobilisation Theory which refers to the processes and practical activities through which actors interpret and create order in conditions of complexity.

Sociomaterial How people's activities shape and are shaped by their use of technologies in a system of work.

Standardisation The specification of 'standards' (rules, guidelines, interventions) to be applied to certain categories of condition, clinical processes or care pathway about the actions that should occur.

Strategic action field Derived from Fligstein and McAdam, the concept of a strategic action field is used in Translational Mobilisation Theory to refer to the contexts in which projects of collective action occur and which furnish the structures, organising logics, interpretative repertoires and materials that condition how an activity is undertaken.

Structures In Translational Mobilisation Theory, structures refer to the patterned elements of a strategic action field that generate the entities, positions and relationships which orient the organisation of an activity.

Technology Medical and surgical procedures, drugs, equipment and facilities and the organisational and supportive systems within which care is provided, including mundane technologies.

Temporal articulation In the Care Trajectory Management Framework, temporal articulation refers to the actions that are taken to ensure activities and events take place at the right time and in the right order.

Tragedy of adaptability This term was introduced to the literature by Wears and Hettinger to refer to how staff workarounds and modifications driven by the desire to accomplish the work can also mask dysfunctional systems; it is the dark side of organisational resilience.

Trajectory articulation Pillar 3 of the Care Trajectory Management Framework, which refers to the material, integrative and temporal articulation of trajectories of care.

Trajectory awareness Pillar 1 of the Care Trajectory Management Framework, which refers to the practices involved in developing and maintaining an understanding of trajectories of care as they evolve.

Trajectory working knowledge Pillar 2 of the Care Trajectory Management Framework, which refers to the practices involved in generating knowledge flows for care trajectory management.

Translation A mechanism in Translational Mobilisation Theory derived from actor network theory, translation refers to the processes that enable practice objects to be shared between participants and their different understandings accommodated.

Translational Mobilisation Theory Developed by Allen and May, Translational Mobilisation Theory is a sociological theory of organisation which describes the relationships between people, materials and technologies in achieving a goal in dynamic systems of work.

Work-as-done A term used in complexity science which recognises that the most powerful organisational processes begin with the staff and their interventions in responding to contingencies in the work environment.

Work-as-imagined A term used in complexity science which refers to idealised understanding of how an activity is accomplished, based on formal organisational processes and plans.

Note: Page numbers followed by '*f*' indicate figures, '*t*' indicate tables and '*b*' indicate boxes.